D1125455

One of *O, The O,*

**"Ten Titles to Pick Up Now"**

. . . . . .

*Acclaim for Susan Conley's*

# The Foremost Good Fortune

"Memoirs, I've come to understand, have a particular way of preparing us. We will all find ourselves up against life-threatening illness, and when we do, the masterful passages in this book will come flooding back to us, bringing perspective and comfort with every remembered word."
— Kelly Corrigan,
author of *The Middle Place*

"It's difficult to move halfway around the world and try to make a home for yourself—even a temporary one—in an alien land. It's harder still to be diagnosed with a serious illness, undergo surgery and treatment, and cope with the aftermath of that process. Undertaking both at the same time seems overwhelming. . . . Conley's ability to describe her challenges honestly, without self-pity, leads you not only to relate to her, but also to admire her."
— *Slate*, "Book of the Week"

"*The Foremost Good Fortune* contains moments both heartwarming and heart-wrenching."
—*The Portland Phoenix*

"I loved this memoir not only for its humor and humility, but for its gentle weaving of disparate elements—dislocation, illness, motherhood, travel, marriage—into a seamless, irresistible whole. It is beautifully written."　　—Monica Wood, author of *Any Bitter Thing*

"Startling, poignant."　　　　　　　　—*More*

"This is an exquisite memoir, a gripping story from page one that tugs you along with the honest questioning and insightful whispers of a courageous best friend." —Jeanne Marie Laskas, author of *Growing Girls*

"Conley's lovely memoir powerfully reminds us that we draw our strength from the many little wonders of our everyday lives."　　—*BookPage*

"Some books pull you into their orbit, taking you to another world. Susan Conley's vivid memoir . . . is a case in point."
—*The Portland Press Herald*

"A story of resilience, told with grace and humor, and with Chinese accents."
—James Fallows, author of *Postcards from Tomorrow Square*

"Rewardingly perceptive and frank."
—*Richmond Times-Dispatch*

"*The Foremost Good Fortune* is told by an intrepid traveler who has found her voice in a daunting, exhilarating cultural wilderness . . . and has found it with wisdom and grace and wonder."
—Michael Paterniti,
author of *Driving Mr. Albert:
A Trip Across America with Einstein's Brain*

"You wouldn't expect to see yourself in Susan Conley's new memoir . . . but you will. . . . A beautifully intimate story of homesickness and culture shock, of motherhood and illness, of China and cancer, and the unwavering truths of family and friends and home."
—*Down East* magazine

"Irresistible. . . . An increasingly metaphysical narrative, Conley's 'travelogue' aptly describes living under Communism, what Beijing was like as it prepared for the 2008 Olympics, and ultimately, what it means to be a foreigner in a strange place."
—*The Post and Courier* (Charleston, SC)

"Far from your typical expat vanity project, *The Foremost Good Fortune* offers surprising depth and clarity on just what it means to live outside our comfort zones." — *The Beijinger*

"Anyone who has ever fallen ill in a foreign country knows how scary that can be. . . . This touching memoir is a study in fortitude and acceptance, an inspiring read with much to say."                                              —*The Missourian*

"Offers insightful glimpses into contemporary China as [Conley] warms towards it, capturing the nuances of Beijing's colorful people and its ancient language and customs amid the country's unrelenting drive toward modernity."
—*Time Out Hong Kong*

"Luminous. . . . Conley's writing is at once spare and strong, and her description of having to present an unflappable front to her children while being hit "with a rolling wave of homesickness" pulls the reader into her world like a close friend."
—*Publishers Weekly* (starred)

SUSAN CONLEY

# The Foremost Good Fortune

Susan Conley lived in Beijing for more than two years, and returned to Portland, Maine, with her husband and two sons in December 2009. She is cofounder and former executive director of the Telling Room, a writers' workshop and literary hub for the region. She was an associate editor at *Ploughshares* and has led creative writing seminars at Emerson College in Boston. Her work has been published in *The New York Times Magazine*, as well as *The Paris Review*, *Harvard Review*, *Ploughshares*, and other literary magazines. She is currently working on her first novel.

www.susanconley.com

# The Foremost
# Good Fortune

# The Foremost Good Fortune

*A Memoir*

## SUSAN CONLEY

*Vintage Books*
*A Division of Random House, Inc.*
*New York*

FIRST VINTAGE BOOKS EDITION, MARCH 2012

*Copyright © 2011 by Susan Conley*

The Library of Congress has cataloged the Knopf edition as follows:
Conley, Susan, [date].
The foremost good fortune / by Susan Conley.—1st ed.
p. cm.
1. Conley, Susan. 2. Conley, Susan—Family.
3. Conley, Susan, 1967– —Health. 4. Beijing (China)—Biography.
5. Beijing (China)—Social life and customs.
6. Americans—China—Beijing—Biography.
7. Cancer—Patients—China—Beijing—Biography.
8. Cancer—Treatment—China—Beijing. 9. Portland (Me.)—Biography.
I. Title.
DS795.23.C66A3 2010
951'.15606092—dc22 [B] 2010036000

**Vintage ISBN: 978-0-307-73986-5**

www.vintagebooks.com

Printed in the United States of America

10  9  8  7  6  5  4  3  2  1

To Tony
and to Aidan and Thorne

Hunger: the foremost illness.
Fabrications: the foremost pain.
For one knowing this truth
As it actually is,
Unbinding
Is the foremost ease.

Freedom from illness: the foremost good fortune.
Contentment: the foremost wealth.
Trust: the foremost kinship.
Unbinding: the foremost ease.

*—translated by Thanissaro Bhikkhu*

# The Foremost
# Good Fortune

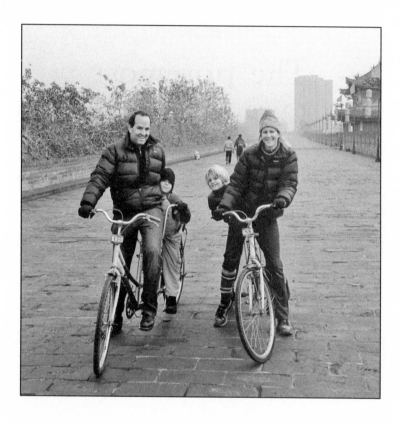

Tony, Susan, Thorne, and Aidan biking on top of the ancient wall of the city of Xian, in Shaanxi Province

# 前门

# Qianmen:
# The Front Gate

It's late on a cold April night in Portland, Maine, and I lie on the couch staring hard at a glossy pullout map of Beijing. My two boys are asleep upstairs in their beds, and my husband has just landed in China to buy swivel chairs for his new office there. I want this map to offer a clue of what a life in Beijing would look like. But the more I gaze at street names, the more distant they feel: would we live on a road called Yongdingmen Xibinhe? Or Changchunqiao?

Tony calls me from the crowded lobby of the Grand Hyatt Beijing. He says the capital city is reinventing itself. There's so much construction, whole streets he once lived on are gone. I pull the map closer and trace one long Chinese highway with my finger while he talks. The black line winds around the city center like a snake. "I can't get a feel," I say out loud and try to laugh into the phone, but the laughter sounds forced. "I'm staring at the Forbidden City. It's smack in the middle of everything, isn't it?"

There's a slight delay on the line—a second of silence that neither of us fills. "It's a city within a city," Tony says. "With shrimp dumplings so good they may change your life." I close my eyes and listen to his voice. I've been hearing China stories from my husband as long as I've known him.

In the eighties he hitchhiked in China for a year on a college grant and became so curious he stopped out for another stay. When I married Tony, I felt China's tidal pull. In San Francisco I pretended to be invested in a legal career, while Tony taught photography at a Chinese community center— walking old men and women around Chinatown, cameras dangling from their necks, and then back to the darkroom he'd built.

We drove to San Diego, where Tony wrote grad papers on Sino-American trade treaties, and I got a master's in poetry. When we migrated to Boston, I taught at a downtown college and Tony put on a consulting tie. But the closest he got to Beijing during the Boston years was our favorite dumpling house. Then we moved to Maine—as far east as we could go in the continental United States. China sat in the rooms of our house like a question.

I can hear Tony say something fast in Mandarin to someone in the hotel lobby. He has what people in China call "pure tones." That means he speaks Chinese almost as if he's lived there all his life. And I don't mean to imply that my husband didn't study his brains out to get a handle on a quadrant of Mandarin's fifty-five thousand characters. But he's good at it in an uncanny way. It's the main reason, really, why I'm still awake at close to midnight, pulling a green wool blanket over my legs, trying to decide if I can transplant my kids to a country where they don't have one friend.

It's time I gave Tony some kind of sign. I've been stalling. There's an apartment lease in Beijing waiting for initials and a work contract that needs negotiating. The question is about geography. But it runs deeper. Given the choice, our two little boys would say they're doing fine, thank you. They are four and six and believe life in Maine means clear oceans and no reason to tinker. No cause to climb on a jumbo jet and fly into the next hemisphere. Or to start over in a new school, in a new city, where they do not speak the language.

No one has to explain to me that the journey will be about confronting unknowns: the nuanced language, and a history so rich that Marco Polo and Genghis Khan both sharpened their teeth there. But also the unknown of the person I've most recently become—a mother still unsure of her new job description. A nap czar and food commandant. Who is *she*? That woman who keeps a pencil drawing of a thermometer taped to the fridge to remind her kids that her temper is rising?

"You haven't asked," is what I finally whisper into the phone.

Tony is confused now. "Asked what?"

"You have to ask me to come to China." I speak louder. "I need you to ask." Then I smile to myself because I am a person guided by words and he is not. But when he starts to talk, I can't detect even a trace of impatience, and that's how I know my answer.

"Okay," he says slowly, and there's a lilt to his voice. "I'm asking if the four of us can move to China." I hear him take an excited breath. "I'm formally asking if you'll come."

That's when I hear myself say yes. Yes to the cultural zeitgeist that living in China the year before the Olympics will surely be. Yes to an exit from the grind of Tony's commuter-flight life. Yes to all the unknowns that will now rain down. Because that one small word sets our family in motion. A month later I resign from the creative writing lab I've been running. We rent out our Portland house and truck old high chairs and baby strollers and frying pans to a storage facility with a corrugated metal roof. Then we ship boxes of rain boots and soccer balls and Early Readers on an airplane to Beijing.

What unfolds in China is the bounty we hoped for: the universe is much bigger once you leave New England. We are meant to grow as a family in that way you hear Americans do when they head east, to become bigger risk takers and deepen our connections to one another. And we do. We eat *jiaozi* and *baozi* and brown, pickled tea eggs. We drive the crooked *hutong* alleys with screaming taxi drivers and climb remote mountains on ancient horses. What's more, the boys and I learn how to speak beginner Mandarin, while Tony dusts off a few vocabulary words.

But what happens while we're there is that one of us gets cancer. It turns out to be me. This is my excuse for why I haven't held on to more Mandarin grammar. For us, cancer becomes the story within the China story. China and cancer are both big countries, so there's a lot to say about each. But let me start back at the beginning. It's Monday in Beijing, and I have to go pick up the boys from their first day of school.

# I

# Hall of
# Celestial and
# Terrestrial
# Union

# 交泰殿

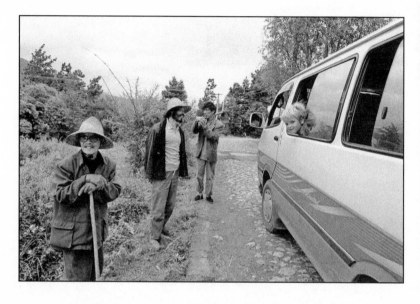

Thorne during a pit stop on a trip through Yunnan Province

# You Should Have Come Earlier

Here's the setup: I'm in the passenger seat of a blue Buick minivan driving through downtown Beijing at three o'clock on a blistering afternoon. A fifty-three-year-old Beijing local named Lao Wu is driving. He will always be the one driving in this story. He wears pressed high-waisted blue jeans and a sharp tan Windbreaker. Driving is his job; that is to say, he's a full-time driver. When Lao Wu came back home from the fields after the Cultural Revolution, the high schools had been closed. That was the week he learned to drive a Mack truck, and he's been driving ever since.

This is my third day in Beijing, and jet lag still pulls me down by my ankles. I lean back in the seat, my mind thick with sleep, and the van slows so I can count twenty waitresses lined up outside the Sichuan Xiao Chi dumpling house. The girls wear blue cotton *qipaos* and do jumping jacks on the sidewalk, then they salute a head waitress who stands on a small, black wooden box. Next they let out a cheer and march in a circle on the sidewalk. The head waitress calls out more instructions (How to fold the napkins? How to take a drink order?) and the girls yell back in a call and response. Then they salute their leader one more time and march into the restaurant.

People don't march much where I'm from. Maybe the

occasional high-school band at the annual Bath Memorial Day parade. But marching is very much the way here—some kind of simulation of the hard-nosed Chinese army way of life? Some kind of leftover from the Communist heyday? Except we're still in the Communist heyday, aren't we?

At the apartment complex where we live there are more marching guards. They salute me every time I come back to the building. It's creepy. I want to tell them I'm not their senior officer. No. I am a forty-year-old American wife and mother of two who can't remember how to pronounce the number *eight* in Mandarin. This is a problem, because eight is where we live. It's China's luckiest number, and let me say right now that numerology is intrinsic to the whole China operation. Numbers here have secret, mystical powers. There are no fourth floors in China because when spoken, the Chinese character for the number 4 sounds too much like the character for death. So what good fortune that our apartment sits on the lucky eighth floor of a building called Park Avenue, across the street from Beijing's biggest city park. It's mostly Chinese families at Park Avenue— well-off Beijingren, the term used for people born and raised in the capital. Many are people who somehow got out during Mao's reign and have returned because China's prospects now look so good. There's also a big handful of Taiwanese here and Hong Kong Chinese and a smattering of Europeans.

We could have lived in Palm Springs or Champagne Villas, Yosemite or Central Park, Park Place or the Beijing Riviera—vast compounds whose names move beyond kitsch into the surreal. To get through the front door of our apartment lobby, we say "Ni hao" to the teenaged guard. He says, "Ni hao" back and salutes us. Then we say "Xie xie," which means thank you, and he says "Bu keqi" (you're welcome), and lets us on the elevator. He salutes us one more time to make sure. We play out this Beckett-like scene of absurdity many times a day, until the humor in it has dried up and flown away on the winds of the Gobi Desert.

Tony has come to introduce credit-rating systems to the Chinese state-owned banks. This means that he meets with senior financial officers, trying to explain in Mandarin why buying complicated American computer programs is crucial to China's success. Sometimes Tony has to pinch himself to make sure it's him and not an imposter wearing that blue banker's suit. Because when Tony lived in Beijing the first time, he had a different gig.

In 1985 Tony took a backpack and a Nikon and headed out on China's trains photographing border zones—places the government here officially calls "ethnic minority regions." Tony started in Yunnan where it meets up with Laos and Burma, and then went northwest to Xinjiang Province where it rubs shoulders with today's "stans": Pakistan, Uzbekistan, Kazakhstan. Next he went south to Tibet and got an early visa for Lhasa. He'd been schooled in Mandarin and had a knack for conversing with strangers, for hitching rides and getting out of pinches with Chinese police. In many towns he was the first *laowai* the locals had seen. He'd arrive in a village and make friends there and find it hard to leave.

Years ago in San Francisco, when it got so I always wanted to be in the same room with Tony, he gave me one of the photos he took on that trip. Some of the prints had won awards in galleries by then. Mine was of two women sitting in a crop of Hami melons by the side of a dusty road. I hung it in my bedroom and it marked the beginning of my own quiet fascination with Asia. The natural beauty of those women startled me, and so did the way they looked right into Tony's camera. The photo made me want to understand him more. He knew himself well. There was a quiet self-sufficiency. Where did that come from?

I have never been to China. I do not speak the language. I've bought a wooden Chinese desk. My plan in Beijing is to finish a novel—two hundred pages of a rough draft set in Paris. The boys are here to go to school. It is what boys do. Or at least that's what I keep telling them they do. Their school is a twenty-minute highway ride south of our apartment. It sits down the road from the underpass that marks one of Beijing's busiest intersections: a six-way juggernaut of rickshaws, one-speeds, VW Santanas, and horses and wagons. Today, a horde of teenage vendors has set up shop on the sidewalks to sell chestnuts and lychees, and baked sweet potatoes. These streets are not pedestrian friendly—they're long blocks of strip malls and food stalls and mid-rises in all stages of rehab and post-hab. Throngs of people walk in the roads buying and selling like mad. There's Tsingtao beer for sale, and turtles, and athletic socks, and phone chargers. How strange and dazzling.

The more I stare, the more arbitrary those marching waitresses back down the road begin to seem—like some kind of imposed order. Finger in the dam. There's so much humanity here; a dozen men take a snooze on the strip of concrete below the overpass. There's a woman walking just ahead in a bright Mickey Mouse T-shirt who pauses to blow her nose into the gutter. To the right of the gridlock, hundreds of people wait in line for buses. A large floral display stands next to the ticket kiosk—something you might see in a Macy's Thanksgiving Day parade, made entirely of yellow chrysanthemums that spell out the words "Beijing 2008 Games." Next to the sign a woman sells slices of yellow Hami melon on wooden skewers. A line of black Audis weaves in front of our van with their lights on and a rose garland battened to each hood. Lao Wu smiles and points to the bride and groom who ride in front of the procession in a blue Hummer.

I've never seen so many people riding bicycles—all helmetless and willing to risk their lives dodging cars. Many women wear black office pumps and knee-length polyester dresses; lots of men are in nylon business slacks with white-collared shirts. At first, the joke would seem to be on the cars, because they can't get through the mess. But it's the cars that will prevail here—one thousand more on the road every day, which makes the bicycles begin to look like living artifacts.

We're creeping through a series of traffic lights, and I'm sure the words I hear on the radio are in English. I ask Lao Wu to turn up the volume by making a circular motion with my right hand. "Ying yu?" I say excitedly. *Is it English?* Then I repeat, "Ying yu?" and then I'm hit with a rolling wave of homesickness.

Lao Wu shakes his head decisively and says, "Han yu." *Chinese.*

But I'm sure I can hear English on the radio. I will it to be English. A motorbike passes—the driver's wife sits behind him with a baby in her lap, and a toddler sits up front on the handlebars. I want to be driving I-95 north from Portland to Phippsburg, listening to the local radio. I want to be sitting in my mother's kitchen in West Point while she reminds my brother, John, on the phone how to make chocolate fudge. John's a very tall man now and one of my best friends, and in the 1970s he made a lot of fudge.

I want to listen to any single conversation I can understand. Because this is too much—an entire country that doesn't speak English. City of fifteen million with no readable road signs. City of marchers. That's when Lao Wu turns up the volume and laughs, and I think I'm going to really like him. I laugh too and nod my head, because of course. Of course it's Chinese on the radio. We are, after all, in China. It's Monday in Beijing and we've got work to do. Children to pick up from school. The first day is bound to be rocky.

We pull up to the school gate, and the street looks like a construction zone: plastic food tubs and paper wrappings line the road. Cement high-rises stretch as far as I can see. Some are empty shells. Others get air-conditioning units soldered by men dangling on ropes. The total sum of so many skyscrapers has a zeroing-out effect. There's such a great deal of heavy machinery and laying of rebar that my mind clouds over.

A green bulldozer barrels through the cars and drops a load of brown dirt to the left of our van. The driver wears a black polyester sports jacket and a yellow hard hat. Ten men attack the dirt with shovels. They're the migrant workers you might have heard about. The ones who've left their farms in the countryside—millions of them—to ready Beijing for the Olympics. They're the ones transforming China. They work for about two dollars a day. The migrant workers don't march. Most of them smoke while they shovel. Some of them are barefoot. Others are shirtless, and theirs is a story of epic migration—of sleeping along this road under green tarps that line the sidewalk, or in flimsy tin barracks behind the work site.

I lean against the metal school gate and look into the court-yard, and that's when the school's security guards leave their posts and begin marching in formation. Their faux-military uniforms—brass belt buckles, long blue jackets, and blue pants—make them look like mid-level army. They march to the open space across from the fleet of parked school buses, where they salute their head guard, which makes me nervous. This is not a military academy, is it? How big a city Beijing must be to hold these contradictions.

The school is called Beijing City International School. We chose it from a Web site. Then Tony took a tour of it when he came over two months ago. The way I see it, this school is a crapshoot. How can you pick teachers from photos on the Internet? The one thing I already like about the place, though, is that few American kids attend. There are Korean children and Taiwanese and Hong Kong Chinese, plus Indians, Australians, Europeans, and Brazilians, but Aidan and Thorne are some of the only Americans in their classroom.

The school advertised a secular curriculum: Chinese language classes every day and a focus on being "internationally minded." There's supposed to be art and music and swimming. No marching. Small people emerge from the building—little children who don't look like they could be old enough to hold their heads up all day. The children's blue backpacks are bigger than their torsos. Here comes Aidan's preschool class. And there's Aidan. He's a thin bean with sandy brown hair and huge almond-shaped eyes. He's usually a dreamer who never stops wondering about the state of the universe. Sometimes he lives entirely in his head. But right now he looks tired and cross, and as soon as he sees me, he starts crying. He thrusts his backpack in my hands. "Do you have a snack for me? Do you have water? I'm thirsty. I'm hot." His teacher, Carmel, is from Australia, and she reminds me of a high-school friend's fun great-aunt. She smiles and tells me warmly that Aidan's had a great first day. She calls him *daaaaarling*. But he won't look at her. She says he's just wound up about getting the answer right in Chinese.

Then Thorne rounds the corner. He's the blond in our family: dark eyes and tan skin and then this shock of bright hair. Thorne likes to be out in front whenever I give up the pole position. He prefers to know the game plan and the score and the names of the opposing players. Thorne and I have telepathy. We're that much alike. Aidan has come to us from another planet, but Thorne is blood of my blood and milk of my milk. Thorne is our camp director. He doesn't have time to dream because he's busy planning the afternoon's aquatic schedule. He doesn't have time to think. I have come to view this as a good thing. And maybe a cunning strategy.

Now he sees me and also shoves his things into my chest: water bottle, backpack, sweatshirt. I can't hold all this stuff, and the water bottle falls. Thorne says, "You should have come earlier. You shouldn't have come to school so late." *But who's late?* I want to ask. If anything, I'm early. "You should have come earlier," he repeats, and then tears start down the sides of his round face and I realize we're in deeper than I thought here. All three of us are overtired. By the time we get to the van, both children have unhinged: Thorne hates his Chinese class and announces he's never going back. "Never," he sobs. "You have no right to make me."

Lao Wu smiles at me uneasily and closes the windows and turns on the AC. He seems as unnerved by the crying as I am and keeps laughing and making tsk-tsk sounds with his tongue as if to quiet Thorne. I smile at Lao Wu, but my hands are shaking a little. I need to talk these boys down. I wonder for a second which tack to take—and exactly how much English Lao Wu can understand. Because it's an odd thing to have your children unravel while a friendly Chinese man you've just met drives you through the Beijing stoplights. What will Lao Wu think of us—these American children and their mother crying their way home from school?

Except I am not crying. Not yet. Crying doesn't feel like an option. There's too much to get right. Aidan drinks from the water bottle I hand him and begins to give me a list of the reasons the new school is terrible. "Really bad," Aidan cries for emphasis. "Small bikes, yucky food. And boring. Boring, boring, boring. Nothing to do."

"Really?" I try not to panic. I look out the window at the passing skyscrapers. Things were good in Maine. And now we've gone and messed with it. I would lie down in this Chinese road for both of my boys, but I can't live in this country with two complainers. I need them to show a little spunk.

"You know why I like my old school better?" Aidan asks.

"No, why?" I say and slightly clench my jaw.

"I like my old school better because it has swings," Aidan explains. "And I wish I were Chinese. Or Korean, because then I would be able to talk to the kids."

"But your new school has swings." I close my eyes for a second. I should state for the record that I have secret mother superpowers. Yes. I have the ability to detach from my children and climb into my own mind at the exact moments my boys might be telling me something they think is vitally important. And I know. I know. It's not necessarily safe. It's not necessarily compassionate. But what I do is build a small room in my head—closet-sized—and go inside and close the door. I can still see them; I just can't quite hear them. I go inside this room so I can think clearly. I go inside because the two boys exhaust me. They never let up. They never go play house or with finger puppets or dolls. They don't even play with Legos. Their games involve running and jumping and leaping off furniture. And they always want me to be the referee. I go inside the room in my mind because it's a way to not blow my top and lose it with them. Before I built this room I used to yell at them more. They were one and three or two and four and always climbing on the small tile ledge around the bathtub. No one was sleeping through the night.

"My old school had sturdier stuff." Aidan sips his water.

"Sturdier?" I look at him closely and wonder about that room in my mind and how quickly I can get in there. Because the machinery in Aidan's head is testing me. His eyes are a shade of brown that looks wet sometimes because the brown is so dark. You can't see the irises. He's four years old—why does his mind spit out words like *sturdier*?

"Yeah." Aidan looks back at me again. "The climbing stuff was sturdier."

Then Thorne chimes in that he doesn't know anyone at this school. "Where are my friends?" It's a simple question. And it deserves a good answer. The boys' urge to belong is palpable. I feel it, too—a primal need to fit in here somehow, to reach some kind of early understanding with China.

By the time we get back to the apartment complex, it's begun to rain. We climb out of the van and say good-bye to Lao Wu. Then one of our Chinese neighbors approaches on the sidewalk and points up to the sky. He's an old man with white hair, and he says in English that each time it rains in Beijing, the temperature drops five degrees. That this is how we get ourselves through autumn in China: rainfall by rainfall, five-degree increments by five-degree increments.

# The Jingkelong

I wake up in my clothes. It's Saturday, and I find the boys and Tony sitting on the floor in our living room (the couch the real estate agent ordered at a nearby factory hasn't come yet). The three of them sweat in the early heat and eat bowls of instant oatmeal I brought from the States. I count over a hundred skyscrapers out the window without turning my head. Tony sees me and jumps up in his blue boxers. "Get your flip-flops on." He smiles. "I'm taking you all for a walk into Old Beijing for breakfast."

I stare at my husband and nod my head slowly—why is he so chipper? I still can't shake the jet lag. Last night I fell asleep in my tank top and sweatpants at six o'clock, facedown on the mattress. It's 7:00 a.m. now, too early to say much of anything, and I force a smile and head down the long hall to our bedroom to change my clothes. September in Beijing is hot. Even with the AC churning, there's no way to outrun the heat.

Our apartment is going to be great—a Chinese take on a Soho loft: high concrete ceilings, large open rooms with empty concrete walls, wood laminate flooring. Tony found it on the same trip that he picked out the school. There's a new kitchen with a dishwasher, an appliance almost unheard-of here two years ago. There's also a washing machine, and a bar with a sink that sits right between the living room and the dining room. I'd seen photos of the place on my laptop but wasn't prepared for the scope—nothing like I'd imagined an apartment in crowded Beijing. "A wet bar?" I had to say to Tony when I first spied it. "You mean like for entertaining?" I asked. "Which would mean a social life?"

The one drawback of the apartment is that it sits on top of one of China's biggest interstates—an eight-lane, full-press freeway called the Fourth Ring Road. This must be the black snake on the map back in Portland. It's a bigger reptile than I imagined and makes noise through the day and the night. I decide we'll buy curtains to cover the windows that face its way, and then we'll never notice it. Aidan and Thorne haven't gotten over the thrill that we live in a building with a real live elevator that we ride every day—one that deposits us into our own small lobby. Our front door opens onto a long concrete corridor—the perfect skateboard alley. It's what sealed the deal for Tony. Because if we have to spend two years hiding out from the Beijing pollution, at least we can play soccer in this hall.

Bedrooms peel off from here—Thorne's is on the right with a double bed and sky blue curtains. Aidan's is on the left: metal bunk beds, green curtains, and enough space to hold a basketball tournament. Tony's and my room sits at the end of the hall. I stand in our walk-in closet and throw on a sleeveless cotton dress, then grab the flip-flops from behind the door. The high ceilings and industrial beige carpet make it almost feel like a conference room in here. From these windows I can look down behind our building: a warren of narrow alleyways and one-room stone buildings. This is an old, tight-knit Beijing neighborhood that Tony calls a hutong. A gaggle of kids kicks a soccer ball in front of a concrete shop that fronts the dirt road.

# The Jingkelong

"Let's go, Sus." Tony opens the front door. "You need to eat something soon to fight the jet lag."

Outside, a small group of men and women is ballroom dancing in black dress shoes next to the stand of poplars in the hutong. Scratchy waltz music plays from a black tape recorder set up under a tree. "Ni hao," Tony calls out. Two of the women smile at him. They look like they're having fun. "Zaoshang hao," he says to two older men pointing bamboo fishing poles into the fetid pond, and they grin. The boys run ahead of us repeating, "Ni hao, ni hao," and do ski jumps in the air. Three of the people in my family seem happy to be here. I'm still one step removed.

When Tony and the boys flew to Beijing, I was teaching an adult poetry course in a tenth-century stone château on the French Riviera. This is the truth. My bedroom overlooked a slice of white beach and the green Mediterranean. At about the time the boys and Tony were rounding the North Pole in their 747, I was taking a dip in a small cove near Cannes. So the boys came to China without me, and I came to China alone, and so far I can't decide if this will be the lasting metaphor for how I experience this country.

Not if Tony has anything to say about it. He's almost giddy with being back. It was no simple thing to orchestrate our move, and he feels the relief of landing us here—work visa and all. He takes my hand and we jog to catch up with the boys, then turn down an alley into a market of food stalls and live animal hutches. There are rabbits for sale and turtles and lots of chickens. A crowd of people moves through the merchandise like a small herd—no lining up. The idea seems to be to shove your way to the front and begin yelling. I hold Aidan's and Thorne's hands tighter, and we stop by a table where Tony manages to buy a dozen brown eggs from a man whose chickens peck at his bare feet.

The chickens make me think of the long talk about avian flu I had with paranoid Dr. Moretti at the vaccination clinic in the States. He said scary things while he gave me the shots, like *The Chinese will always be watching you. They'll always know where you are.* And other slightly more sane things, like *Don't go to chicken farms in China. Don't pet the chickens.* But Tony is shining today. It's as if he's been waiting for this morning for twenty years. He has Aidan's brown hair and the same big, almond-shaped eyes, and he can't stop smiling.

The sky is blue and so clear, I can see the ring of sloped mountains beyond the city. From here they look earth-colored and inviting. Maybe they got the air pollution thing in China all wrong. Great big rafts of cumulus float by, and the sun shines on the tall willows in the park beyond. We pass a stall selling pink carnations and sunflowers and then a shop with a sign in English that reads "Adult Health: Bondage Toys." The rest of the signage on the street is in Chinese characters, and when I look at these signs I end up feeling like I've dropped down into some Asian netherworld. Some essential Beijing at the epicenter of China. Tony raises his eyebrows at the sex shop and we keep walking toward a dumpling place we've heard about. We pass five stalls with open woks set up on the sidewalk. The plastic tables are different colors—yellow and green and turquoise—and come up to my shins. The stools are smaller; adults perch on half their bottoms, slurping noodles from white bowls.

The smell is of garbage and open sewage and garlic. A kind of Chinese Muzak blares from one vendor's transistor, and all that marching of waitresses and security guards I saw on Monday feels like a memory. Like it masks the real China, which might be here in the two straw baskets of fresh chestnuts a man balances off his shoulders from a wooden yoke. He would like me to buy some. "Bu yao xie xie," I say to him, relieved that I've already memorized the phrase for what I don't want in this country.

We sit at one of the round tables fit for preschoolers, and Tony calls out for the waiter. Everywhere we go in Beijing there's an epidemic of soft drink consumption, and now the boys beg for Cokes. We're breaking the rules from home, and it's exhilarating. "Fuwuyuan," Tony yells again. And then louder. I cringe at my husband's moment of American imperialism—he's usually so low-key. That's when Tony tells me that the only way to get a waiter in China is to yell. There are no menus, and what you do is get the attention of someone who looks like they work here, and ask them what's good to eat. "They won't come until you scream, Sus. It's the custom."

Sure enough a teenage boy jogs over, and he and Tony begin a shouting match about which dumplings are best and if there are some with shrimp, not pork. Aidan hears the word *shui,* which means water. "Sprite, at least," he begs. "If we can't have Coke then at least Sprite." I look at Tony and am perfectly willing to give in to Sprite for breakfast. I'm tired, and everything here is open for bargaining.

It's a heady feeling to think we're going to live in this city for at least two years. Where will we buy toothpaste? How will we find a way to feel like we belong? I want to mark this moment somehow—the four of us sitting in the alleyway for the first time, waiting for dumplings. Because time is already moving ahead; I can feel it. Winds of change are sweeping through Beijing while we decide whether to have soda for breakfast. It's hot in this alleyway and I have a headache coming on. "Give them soda," I say to Tony. "Soda will be our friend this morning."

A circle of men in their twenties huddle around the table next to us, and when they finish their dumplings, they all light up cigarettes. I look around and most everyone else out here is smoking if they're not eating. Some are doing both. This is when Thorne begins to worry. "The smoking," he says. "It's making me sick." I try to brush it off. I say they do smoke a lot of cigarettes in China. "But they're killing themselves," Thorne explains. Which is the mantra we've always told the boys, who think of cigarettes as something close to heroin.

Maybe this kind of schooling is a mistake, because now Thorne gets up from the table and storms away. Tony runs after him. Thorne must be trying to piece it together—how it is we came to be here, and what we're going to do with our days. But I'm projecting. I'm often guilty of that. Maybe it's me who's trying to figure out where we've landed.

Aidan puts his head in my lap and begins to count in Chinese. If you can get from one to ten in Mandarin, then you're on your way to one hundred. The numbers seem to make Aidan's brain feel good. Aidan already has the purest Mandarin tones of any of us. Tony says it's because he's the youngest. I can't make the sounds Aidan makes in Chinese. He's laughing and gets to fifty-five (*wu shi wu*). *Wu* is pronounced almost like *wooooooo*. Aidan says it perfectly, cutting it off the way you'd stop a horse: *whoa*.

"You're the new smoking police," I tell Thorne when he sits back down. "From now on you can give out citations."

"What is a citation?" he asks, and takes a drink of Sprite.

"A ticket," Tony says. "You can write up smoking tickets and hand them out on the street to anyone you see smoking." Thorne laughs, and then the dumplings come and they're boiled, not steamed or fried, and a little doughy on the outside and delicious. We dip them in a round dish of soy sauce and vinegar that sits on the table, and our little ship is righted again.

. . .

After the dumplings, I feel emboldened. I leave the boys with Tony at a small bike shop and head over to the Jingkelong that sits at the end of the main street. It's time to do a little retail work. For starters, I need apples. There were no apples in the hutong market. I also need a hair dryer. My requirements for this are simple: the dryer needs to be able to dry my hair. Until now I've air-dried and then tied it up in a black elastic and forgotten about it.

The Jingkelong is big (think Costco or Walmart) and intimidating. It's filled with lots of people speaking fast Chinese, plus four whole floors of live carp and bulk rice and woks. There are so many people in here I could get lost in the appliance aisle, and Tony would never find me. I stand on the third floor and shyly motion to one of the uniformed clerks, who reaches for the hair dryer I point to. But she doesn't give it to me. She writes out a receipt and waves me to a cashier, who takes the slip and makes copies of it in triplicate.

I think capitalism smells different here. It's old-school. They hardly ever use credit cards. Instead we walk around with big wads of cash. Still, it looks as if everyone's buying things like mad at the Jingkelong. It just takes longer. Money is a bigger deal. That's what happens, I think, when you still have nine hundred million peasants living on the equivalent of less than five U.S. dollars a day. The transaction gets scrutinized.

After the cashier hands me one of the receipts, I'm led to another cashier (they're all wearing matching blue polyester pantsuits) at another counter, where I'm supposed to come up with eighty-five yuan (about twelve U.S. dollars). I hand over the money, and she gives me a different receipt—something to document the sale, maybe. Then I pass both receipts to a runner, who heads to a stockroom, then reappears carrying my hair dryer. This has all taken almost three-quarters of an hour.

On my way to the produce section, I see turtles swimming in cloudy tanks, shells big as Frisbees. Dark eels float nearby. In the cleaning products aisle, different salesgirls are dressed up in costumes: short red skirts and matching jackets and high, shiny red boots. One girl tries to sell me a new kind of synthetic floor mop. She wears her microphone on a headset and calls to me in Chinese to come watch the demonstration where she takes off the mop head and washes it.

Who knew supermarkets could become impromptu talent shows? There's the man who wants me to watch him fry an egg in a Teflon wok, and then the teenage girl further down who's calling to me to watch her use a bagless vacuum cleaner. I make it to apples. I would like to buy a dozen to keep in a bowl on my new kitchen counter. The boys have been asking for apples all week. There's an old man looking at the oranges who has a small bird in his jacket pocket. I can hear it chirping. I grab a plastic bag and fill it with apples. I fill another bag with pears because they look so ripe. Then I head to the row of cash registers. I have my hair dryer in one hand and the fruit in the other. Things have taken so long I've given up on the salt I need. But the teenage cashier wants nothing to do with my fruit. She keeps pointing to the back of the store—way, way back to some hinterland where they must have a scale that I won't know how to use because the directions are in Chinese.

I smile at the checkout girl. I will her to show a little empathy—to see that I'm reaching here. Stretching. I'm going to learn more of the language, but for now I need this nice checkout girl to ask some other nice person to help me weigh my apples and pears. But the girl does not smile back. She stares, and the look is hard and impassive. She tells me something fast again—something that sounds mean and important. Probably about how I'm wasting her time and would I please go weigh my apples myself.

More people stare. I would stare at me too—flustered foreigner with a big bag of unweighed apples. I think I'm closing in on my first public Beijing cry. And so I walk. I leave the apples and pears in their clear plastic bags on the metal checkout counter. Soon I'm just a figment of the checkout girl's imagination—I'm at the automatic doors and then I'm back on the hot sidewalk with the motor scooters and rickshaws. I'm thinking China is relentless.

At dinner Tony and I do a speed-talking test because the Jingkelong has thrown me. Maybe if that checkout girl had spoken a little more slowly this morning, I could have pieced things together. Tony loves to speak Chinese at home—so much, in fact, that he's turned dinnertime into a Mandarin-only game, which the boys think is great. So tonight the four of us speak in Chinese monosyllables and eat the spaghetti I've made for the second night in a row. Aidan passes Thorne a piece of bread and says, "Yao bu yao?," slang for *Do you want it?*

Thorne says, "Bu yao, bu yao" (*Don't want*), and laughs. They seem to be catching on quickly.

I'd like to see if Mandarin really is spoken faster than English or if it's just my imagination, so Tony says, "Ni hao, ni ji dian hui jia?" (*Hello, what time are you going home?*) at what I would consider average-speed Mandarin, and I time him: two seconds. Then he says the same sentence as fast as he can in English: three seconds. To me it sounds like gibberish. I conclude from this in-depth analysis that what I've suspected is true: Chinese people really do talk faster than Americans, and this is why I can never understand what's being said in this country.

·　·　·

On Sunday morning we head to the mountains in the van with Lao Wu. The idea is to drive to the base of a small range northeast of Beijing, where we'll hike two hours to an old Buddhist temple. I sit in the front seat and try out my limited vocabulary. I bet this makes Tony wince—my tones are wrong—but I've got to start someplace and stop relying on Tony to do the talking for me. I haven't found a Chinese teacher yet, and each day I try to poach Aidan and Thorne's school vocabulary words.

My favorite new word is *keyi*. I've learned that *keyi* generally means okay—as in, everything is okeydokey. I believe, perhaps falsely, that Chinese people are less irritated with my mixed-up Mandarin when I use the word *keyi*. I ask Lao Wu how his health is in Chinese—it's one of the first sentences I've learned. He tells me things are keyi. I think things are always keyi for him. Or he makes them keyi. The English translation of Lao Wu is "elder Mr. Wu." To call him Lao Wu is to follow the Chinese custom of showing respect to the father.

Lao Wu is that calm, capable Beijing man who is pure keyi. You would want this man driving your kids around the back alleys of Beijing. He is my new favorite Chinese uncle. Then he raises his finger above the steering wheel like an orchestra conductor and shows me the up-and-down intonations for the four tones: 1, 2, 3, 4: ma¯, má, ma, mà. The language lends itself to a bluntness I haven't gotten used to yet. We talk about the weather. "Rain?" I ask him in Mandarin. "Mei you," he answers, which means no rain. "Wind?" "Jin tian mei you. Ming tian you." Which means "No wind today. Tomorrow big wind." Then Tony translates while Lao Wu tells us about the price of chestnuts (high) and the state of Chinese relations with Japan (not so good). When Lao Wu isn't driving he says he's cooking—large Chinese feasts of jiaozi and handmade knife noodles for his wife and their adult twins, Xiao Wu (little Wu) and Wei Wang, and their spouses.

I look through the windshield and watch the clusters of high-rises begin to thin. The boys sing a new song, called "Peng you." Tony says it's about a search for a friend at school. Lao Wu begins to sing with them. I have a hope this morning that in leaving Beijing, I might gain distance on the place—some purchase on the city—a clue how it got so big. People say Beijing is an unlikely place for a capital city; the land is dry and flat and abuts the desert. The trees out here seem to have been felled in the previous century and then replanted last week in a massive reforestation project after the sandstorms had already scoured the soil. Hundreds of thousands of short, thin trunks dot the landscape—poplars and willows and cypress.

I turn and ask Tony if Lao Wu has siblings. I can't help but see Lao Wu as one small China frame of reference. It turns out he's a firstborn son, the fourth of five siblings whom he didn't see for years during the Cultural Revolution. He tells Tony that when he was sixteen he was "sent down" to live on a farm with peasants in the countryside for three years. Every day others died around him. He says he figured out how to forage for food on the farm—looking in the same overturned potato fields each day.

I tell him this must have been very difficult, *hen nan*. I'm grateful I know this small Chinese phrase, though in any language my words would be lacking. Would be insufficient. But I need to say something to show him how hard I've been listening. Lao Wu doesn't dwell. He laughs and looks in the rearview mirror and begins teaching the boys a Chinese tongue twister about fourteen stone Chinese lions. We pass a tanker truck covered in a brown tarp, and Lao Wu tells us he used to drive a truck as big as that. Aidan and Thorne keep pointing at the road. "Did you drive one as high as that truck? Or that one?" Thorne demands. "Or what about that one over there?"

Lao Wu is measured. He doesn't drive fast. He explains to Tony that the government has installed a series of video cameras along the highway that record your speed. When there's a lot of traffic, Lao Wu goes into something I'll call "the trance." There's so much information coming at him from the street—rickshaws and motorbikes and passels of pedestrians huddled to cross without getting hit—that he stops speaking and his face becomes still, almost as if he's pulled a mask over it. Just his eyes move.

We take a sharp right and head up into mountains shrouded in mist like on Chinese postcards I've seen. Or is that smog instead of mist? Dry crop beds line the road, and dark yellow corn roasts in the sun next to piles of bricks. The boys wrestle and then Tony puts Aidan in the seat belt next to him, tells Thorne to take a five-minute time-out in the back, and hands out pieces of chewing gum.

We pass a flock of sheep next to the side of the road. Some are sheared and others still have matted wool coats. The old man tending them wears a straw hat and flip-flops. There's a truck at the intersection with two fat pigs in the back behind iron gates. The mountains look greener the closer we get. Aidan has to pee, and there's nowhere to stop, so Tony finally has him go in a water bottle he holds for him in the backseat. Thorne thinks it's hilarious and laughs so hard he cries, and then he has to go in the bottle too.

There are no houses now, just peach trees. Tony translates a sign that reads "Welcome to the largest peach village under the heavens." A gigantic plastic peach sits on a boulder. I feel for a moment like Tony and I are on the great China road trip we used to dream about fifteen years ago in San Francisco. Except now there are two small boys in the back of the van begging for apple juice. Who are those children? And where are their parents?

When we first got married, Tony and I took trips from California in his Toyota pickup—to New Mexico, Baja, Colorado, Idaho. We traveled up to Canada and down through Washington State and Oregon, then over to Arizona. We found excuses to drive anywhere we could, and my life felt to me then like something exciting and vaguely infinite. Now we pass hundreds of peach farmers bartering by the side of the road. Traffic snarls. Some of the trucks stop in the middle and farmers get out to eye the competition. We drive slowly around them. "Who knew," I say to the boys, "that we were going to the peach capital today?" Then Lao Wu begins to teach the boys a song that Tony says is about the twelve different animals in the Chinese lunar cycle.

We park next to a food kiosk that marks the path up to the temple. There's a man at a table selling aluminum cooking pots and bike tires and a stall next to it with bamboo baskets full of red bean baozi. Tony buys two of the rolls for the boys. A man has fallen asleep on peach crates stacked next to the bike tires. Thorne stands next to him and points to a painting on the side of what must be the local school: a Chinese Snow White and her seven dwarfs.

We begin to climb the stone stairs carved into the mountainside. At first Aidan has nothing in his legs, and I have to pull him by his arm. I'm tired and thirsty and getting crankier. The path is not auspicious: it's lined with pieces of toilet paper and empty potato chip bags. Tony is on me about studying Mandarin. "When will you start? Have you made any inroads with teachers? Any traction at all?"

I don't answer because he's been asking this for days—all week, really. Then I say, "I will. I will learn Chinese. We only just got here so can't we leave it alone?" It hits me again that we've moved so far away from our friends and family as to be unreachable. We only have each other in China. What kind of life is that going to be?

On the Monday before I left for China, I had an appointment with an astrologer named Brie in a small, wooden house in Maine. My friend Lily had given me the session as a part-ing birthday gift. She and I share an astrological sign—we're both Cancers. Crabs. Born in the month of July, we carry our houses on our backs. Lily thought an astrology session was the send-off I needed—a way to get some perspective on how my little family might fare in the larger cosmic universe.

Lily is a writer. She's published three novels mapping the fragile ecosystems of families. Brie's reading of her chart that summer made Lily feel she was on exactly the right creative path, doing precisely what the stars had determined for her on the day of her birth. So I figured Lily understood this astrol-ogy thing. "Besides," she yelled as I backed my car out of her driveway and headed off to Brie's, "having your chart read is fun! You'll love it!"

I sat in Brie's house the day before my flight, listening to the alarming news that I'd come into this lifetime carry-ing a cosmic wound. "Don't worry," she assured me. "We all carry this scar." Brie was a sunny, compact woman with strawberry-blond hair and a round face. Her daughter played outside in a sandbox. Brie said we'd all lived on this planet many times before. Then she told me, "Your chart shows Sat-urn squared to Mercury." I nodded. I had no idea what she was talking about.

Brie explained I am partly ruled by Saturn, which is not conducive to a writing life. "Saturn will *want* to try to take over your creative mind," Brie explained, as if this were a completely reasonable way to consider my future. There was hope, she said. Neptune. But only if I vanquished Saturn. I sat baffled—unnerved by the cosmic battle shaping up. And this was a *gift* from Lily? I laughed out loud, and Brie eyed me oddly. "Saturn is all about order." Brie seemed kind of excited now. "And don't think moving to China is going to automatically make you closer to Tony," she warned. I leaned back on her small white couch and tried to resist the urge to flee. She said I was going to have to embrace Neptune to get what I wanted in my marriage and in my writing. I wondered what was wrong with this woman, giving me such heavy news on the eve of my flight.

Halfway up the mountain, the boys find their legs and begin to race. They put each other in headlocks and pour water down their foreheads from their water bottles. It takes us two hours to get to the top. Down below are the peach trees of China. The tiny villages stretch out like connect-the-dots back toward the highway. My life begins to look more finite the longer I stand there. It's a sensation that has to do with the passage of time—the series of choices that landed me north of Beijing, with two boys and a husband, on the top of this green mountain.

The temple is small and square, and Tony translates the carved wooden sign above the door for us: "Welcome to this holiest of shrines. Pray your sickness away." There was a time right after college when I was lucky enough to go to Asia. My grandfather had died that year. He was not a rich man, but a generous one, with a giant laugh. He wore silver wire spectacles and had croppings of white hair around his bald head. He lived for the tomatoes he grew in his gardens and any history of John Adams he could get his hands on. He wore flannel shirts buttoned to the top in high summer and called his wife of sixty years "the Madame." He died of heartbreak months after she did and left each of his children a small sum of money. When my mother gave part of hers to my brother and sister and me, she decreed that we had to travel on it. She knew the good that came from packing a bag and hitting the road. So that was the deal. In 1990 two thousand dollars went a long way in dive hotels of India, Thailand, and Indonesia.

So I have been inside temples. But never with Tony. Never with the boys. And I am not a religious person. The surprise of finding ourselves standing in this dark stone temple with the smell of burning incense is not lost on me. There's a monk who never stops chanting—he tilts his head slightly toward us when we step inside and keeps banging a small drum in his lap with two sticks. It's a high-pitched roving song he sings. I look up and there's a gold Buddha staring down at us. Peaches and coins sit on the table below him. I watch Tony slip to his knees on one of the yellow prayer pillows. A Chinese man kneels next to him with burning incense sticks in each hand. He holds them up to the Buddha and then raises his head and begins reciting a prayer. The boys drop to their knees and lean their small bodies toward the floor. How do they know how to do this?

I kneel down too. It's been so long since I've prayed. When I was growing up, our farmhouse sat down a long dirt drive-way at the edge of a field. On Sunday mornings we'd watch cartoons and chop wood or feed the sheep. Then my father would drive my brother and sister and me to Ron's Superette for the newspapers and Sky Bars. My dad is a third-generation Mainer by way of County Cork, Ireland. He grew up sitting in mass and resigned from church when he turned eighteen. My mother comes from a tribe of Welsh and French Episcopalians. More than religion, what consumed many of her people was music and how to better teach the deaf. My mother has played the oboe since she was young, and it was the hymns that drew her out every few Sundays to church. She said singing hymns with a real organist—uplifting hymns, not those somber dirges, mind you—was as good a way to get a handle on your life as any.

But no one was doing any praying in our house. At least not that I was aware of. I tried praying for a month in junior high because my friends were doing it. But I'm not sure I can call the wish making I did then "really" prayer. Tony is the religious one in our family. He would say no, not religious, but Daoist, maybe, after the years he's spent studying ancient Chinese philosophy. What I've been able to figure out about Daoism in the years I've been married to Tony is that there's one big river we're all swimming in. The trick, Tony explains, is to not fight the current. To let the river carry you.

So I kneel next to Tony in the temple at the top of the mountain, and I close my eyes and thank the Buddha for our health—for the boys' hard little legs and stomachs. Then I wonder if the Buddha can help steady us. Steady me. Because I'm feeling a little wobbly in China. There's another man with his eyes closed in a chair behind the altar. I only see him after I've prayed. When I rise from the floor, he rings a brass bell, and it makes a sweet sound that seals in my prayer. It feels like something has been consecrated inside the temple. Like maybe in China I'll finally learn to give up some control and let the river take me.

Aidan and Thorne are outside, staring at a lime green praying mantis perched on the top of a broom handle. Aidan can't get over it. He's so excited he asks me if the mantis was once a person and I say, "Yeah, maybe."

"Because it looks like a little man, Mommy. A little man praying."

"What if there were no humans?" Thorne asks Tony. "Just insects."

"It would be a very different world." Tony hands each of them a pretzel from his stash. "You never know," he says. "If you're Buddhist, then this mantis is a person. A small, bright green person, praying."

"Maybe Buddhism is for you, Thorne," I say. "Buddhists believe you come back to this world for many different lifetimes."

At home in the States we never talked about reincarnation. I take a sip of water and look closely at my children, then down at the green valley below. At home we never prayed. How is it my boys were so quick to get down on their knees inside the temple?

"Maybe I'll come back next time as a praying mantis," Thorne decides. "Can I? A bright green mantis who rubs his front legs together?"

# The Great Wall Is Older Than Johnny Cash

The next week is when Thorne starts singing. It's early September and he walks around the apartment belting out songs in falsetto. I'm trying not to worry. But now that I've noticed, it seems like he sings all the time—during breakfast yesterday morning and while we played Monopoly after school. He can't seem to stop. He mostly sings patriotic American songs—"America the Beautiful" and "The Battle Hymn of the Republic"—which makes it weirder.

Thorne's first-grade teacher, Diba, is calling the singing a delayed response to moving to China—part of the same "spillover stress." Today Thorne repeated the opening of the national anthem at least fifteen times at breakfast: "O! say can you see by the dawn's early light."

It's like watching an involuntary tic. He has different registers for different songs—he also sings with a vibrato and in a wavering operatic soprano. We can't get him to stop. Except it has to stop. Because it's driving me crazy. Tony cooks a stir-fry in the wok he's brought from the States. He finds it relaxing to slice garlic and chop broccoli florets. Tonight he mixes chunks of ginger with lime juice, then adds coriander and fresh pumpkin. "Try this." He reaches a spoon toward my mouth while I fill the water glasses. "Come on. You'll love it."

And he's right. It always amazes me how much pleasure Tony gets from feeding people, whether it's a dinner for three or twenty. We've always shared the cooking. Sometimes I love to cook. Other times I do it because I have to. Tony cooks because he enjoys it. We sit at the wooden dining table and Thorne sings "Kumbaya" over and over: "Someone's singing, Lord, kumbaya." His voice echoes, even with the red Tibetan rug I've hung on the wall. We try to eat the rice and vegetables, but Thorne keeps singing. So Tony and I make a rule. We say it's too distracting to hear songs while we eat. Thorne doesn't take it hard when we ask him to zip it. Not that he really can stop. He just gets quiet and has a sip of water. Then he announces nervously, "Here we are in China," and starts to hum "This Land Is Your Land."

Aidan has turned to music in a different way. For Aidan there's one song. And one man. His name is Johnny Cash. Aidan has been playing "Ring of Fire" over and over for days. Today I put in a salsa CD just before dinner, then Aidan slipped Johnny back in. I slid in Van Morrison, but by the time dinner was finished, Aidan had won again.

What he does is press the button on the CD player until he reaches song number fifteen. Then that upbeat tempo kicks in. It's like a marching band at first, then it moves into mariachi: "Love is a burning thing . . ." Aidan cannot get enough. He sings along to every word: "I fell into a burning ring of fire. I went down, down, down and the flames went higher." Just before bedtime I hear the song again. I walk into the living room to find my son lying facedown on the floor near the speaker. "What is a ring of fire, Mom? And did it burn him? Did it burn Johnny?"

I deliberate for six seconds, then I say, "Johnny Cash was having a hard time in his life. He was in love. He was not in a ring of actual fire."

"So he was not burning? Johnny Cash's life was not on fire?"

"No," I say and pick Aidan up off the floor and carry him to bed.

"Will you stay with me?" he asks. He's been angling for this every night since we got here. "I don't like to be alone."

Aidan sleeps on the bottom bunk in his room. Often this month I've given in and climbed up the narrow ladder around midnight and crawled under the blankets. He always says he just wants to know I'm there. During the daytime he and Thorne hit tennis balls in here and kick drop shots against the concrete walls. It's the nighttime that gets to Aidan, when his room morphs into a dark zone he doesn't recognize. "I'll check on you in a half hour," I say, and kiss him on the forehead. "Good night, my sweet." He opens his arms for one last hug. I leave without daring to ask if he feels like his own life is burning.

On the weekend we drive north with Lao Wu—this time two hours to a small Tibetan-run ranch near the Great Wall. Thorne is still singing. In the car he remembers almost all the words to "American Pie." Aidan joins, and then Tony and I. It's a funny thing to sing this long American anthem to rock and roll while Lao Wu stares at the China road.

The ranch is a curious mix of old Tibet meets Manchurian cowboy. The staff wears long, traditional Tibetan silk robes. Antique riding saddles and swords hang on the walls. There's a stagnant river outside our small guesthouse. The long-haired Tibetan teenager at the front desk says the water used to be full of wild trout. Four vicious dogs stand tied to trees along the path to our room. They look like wolves, and I think they'll kill us if they break free. Each time we pass, they lunge and bare their fangs and I scream. I want to say something to the other Tibetan teenagers who seem to run this place about the dogs. Something along the lines of, *Are you out of your minds to keep wild wolves at a hotel?* But I could never speak that many words in Chinese and Tony thinks we might want to play it safe. Don't want to get on anyone's bad side at a place with attack dogs. Besides, he says, he knows this kind of Tibetan mastiff, and they're mostly all talk, though he once got terrorized by one on the outskirts of Lhasa.

We make it past the wolves and into our room. "Back then," Tony explains as he opens the front door, "when I traveled in China there were so few foreigners."

"Tell us where you went again?" I bend to take off my sneakers. I've heard these stories before, but Thorne and Aidan haven't. "Where exactly did you hitchhike?" The room is taken up by the *kang,* a giant Chinese bed of bricks built into the wall, where the entire family—mother, father, in-laws, and children—slept head to toe. And when it was cold in the unheated house a fire was lit underneath.

We lie down together on the kang. "I hitchhiked overland in Tibet from Lhasa to a town called Ali, along the Indian border," Tony says with his eyes closed.

"India!" Thorne pops his head out from under the red quilt. "I know where India is on the map."

"So I spent nine days crossing the plateau on the gearshift of a gigantic Japanese truck, driven by a chain-smoking madman delivering a huge load of lumber. Ali has a strategic spot on the border and China wanted to build the town up from nothing."

"Nine days?" Thorne asks. "Sitting in between the two front seats?"

"Nine. There were five of us in the cab. We'd sleep outside at night."

"Tell them the part about the policeman." I roll over to my side. It's cold on the kang, even under the blankets.

"Police?" Aidan says and looks over. Until now he's been staring at the ceiling, deep in thought, perhaps listening. Perhaps not. But he's fascinated by police—by anything to do with rules and punishment.

"We finally got to Ali," Tony continues, "and I went to sleep in a guesthouse but then the police busted in and woke me up and brought me to the station." Aidan looks wide-eyed. "At first," Tony says, "the police weren't nice."

"Oh no!" Aidan calls out.

Thorne laughs out loud. He does that when he's nervous. "They told me I was in a place foreigners shouldn't go. They were mad. But then"—Tony props his head up on his elbow—"the police decided to take me to dinner."

"Dinner?" Aidan can't believe it. "So they were not mad anymore?"

"No. Especially," Tony turns to me and says, "after they plied me with *baijiu* [a kind of Chinese grappa] and got me to tell them about Cyndi Lauper. Then they put me on a bus to Kashgar."

I have this new image in my head of my husband as a twenty-year-old, six-foot, brown-haired backpacker winning over the local security. Here he *wants* to talk to strangers. In the States he was more reticent.

In Boston he'd come alive in a cramped Chinese restaurant called Wings. It was a basement place on a busy Chinatown corner, and the food became Tony's conduit to the mainland. I didn't know the names of China's provinces then; I just knew what tasted delicious. We lived in Boston for seven years. Tony became friends with the owner, Mr. Wong, and his wife, who did most of the cooking. Each time we stepped down into the drop-ceilinged dining room, Tony transformed into a chatterbox—a man who could debate the finer qualities of braised eggplant with Mr. Wong in Mandarin with a rapturous look on his face.

My husband stayed close to his parents after their divorce. His mother is a designer who lives on an island in Maine now. His father made a life as a marble sculptor with Tony's stepmother in New Hampshire. Tony has a track team of nine combined siblings and a posse of friends across the States, but in 1985 he thought nothing of going off the grid in China's mountains alone for months.

Tony sits up quickly in the kang and grabs Aidan's ankle and starts tickling his toes until Aidan screams, he's laughing so hard. Then Thorne joins in and they wrestle until Tony crawls back under the quilt. "I give up!"

"What did you do in Kashgar?" I ask. I still find it hard to understand how he got around—how he lived on the road without a plan.

"There was this group of older, bearded Muslim men there who tended their gardens in the mornings and talked to me while they smoked in the shade in the afternoons. They were Uighurs. They wanted to hear about the rest of the world. To hear about America," Tony explains. I try to imagine my husband sitting in a Uighur courtyard talking to the elders about the beaches of California.


Behind our guesthouse is a sign directing us to the Great Wall with a carved arrow that looks like it points straight up the cliff. Tony and Thorne leave to climb, and I convince Aidan to stay on the ground. He is only four years old, after all—two whole years younger than Thorne. Aidan and I walk to the outdoor dining room for milk tea and a bowl of delicious vanilla yogurt they serve here with golden raisins from the mountain. We sip our tea and watch a scraggly white duck paddle in what's left of the river. "Why can't the duck fly?" Aidan asks.

"It's been clipped," I explain. "Someone has cut one of its wings just enough so it can't take off."

The Tibetan waitress smiles when I ask her where the fish have gone. She tells me in English that the restaurants in Huairou mostly farm their trout in freshwater concrete pools. She's eighteen, on a work visa from Tibet. She misses her family, she says. Soon the ranch will close for the winter. It's already almost too cold to stay in the unheated rooms. Then, she explains, she'll take a train for four days across China, back up into the Tibetan plateau, where her people are from.

She leaves to begin chopping garlic and ginger for dinner. I ask Aidan what he likes most about China so far. He says he likes some of the boys he's met. "The older boys." And by that he means Thorne's six-year-old friends. "But I liked the sleeping better in Portland." "The sleeping," as we have come to call it, remains tricky. Aidan still wakes up every night with a complaint: new noises, he's too thirsty, needs water. He's unsettled.

"How great is it that you already have friends here?" I ask him. "How great is China?" He eyes me with a steady, noncommittal gaze, and then takes a sip of tea. I look down at the menu. "When Thorne and Daddy get back," I say, "we can choose yak or venison or Mongolian beef for dinner."

"But not fish," Aidan reminds me. "We won't have fish, because there aren't any left."


In the morning, we take a taxi to the Great Wall, and Thorne hums the melody to the Erie Canal song. The funny thing about his singing is that sometimes when I recognize the tune,

I can't help but join in. So I sing, "Low bridge, everybody down. Low bridge for we're coming to a town." Then we wait in line for the cable cars. A crowd of Chinese tourists swells behind us, and when the cable finally starts up, we become part of a small, inexplicable stampede. I try to hold Thorne's hand but lose him in the rush at the turnstile, and he calls out my name until I squeeze around a dozen bodies and grab him by the arm. A line of empty cable cars sits waiting for us. I want to yell at the crowd, "What is wrong with you people? Can't you see there are enough for all of us?"

We slide into a car, and three middle-aged Chinese join us: a man and his wife and their female friend. The two women examine our clothes and our shoes and our hair. When they decide they approve, the smiles come. Then they insist on taking our picture and get bossy. "Move," they urge us in Chinese. One holds the camera close to her eye and shoots. "Move closer together."

When we get to the wall, we're quiet at first. I am not sure how to approach the wall. How to *be* on it. Do we walk normally? Slowly? Do we touch the stones? Sit down on the sides? It's so compelling, this wall and its geometry. And so overwhelming. It may be the scope—it stretches up and over the mountains as far as I can see—but this wall asks you to relinquish your hold on things. To give up the reins. We're speechless for whole minutes, and then the four of us are running and jumping and taking hundreds of pictures. It's stunning up here—rural China spreads out below for miles, sun-drenched and russet-toned. We eat soft baozi rolls and cold eggs from a picnic bag the cook at the ranch packed.

From this vantage everything on the wall feels ancient and sacred—even the old men peddling cheap plastic flags. The boys say they'd like to live up here. In tents. And keep watch for Mongol warriors. Then Tony tells them that an emperor from the Ming dynasty oversaw the building of most of this stretch of wall we're on. Aidan asks how long ago this Ming emperor died. "Hundreds of years ago." Tony stops to take a picture.

"So this wall was built before Johnny Cash died?" Aidan wonders.

I look down at my son, and he's not joking. Should I be worried? Who knew how far "Ring of Fire" was going to take Aidan. "The Great Wall," I say slowly, "is ancient, Aidey." Then I smile at him and take his hand.

"So that's good," Aidan decides. "That means this is a very old place. That means the Great Wall of China is older than Johnny Cash."

# Building a Chinese Boat

On the Monday after we get back, my new Chinese teacher, Rose, arrives and says I should think of learning Chinese like trying to build a boat—a long and deliberate process. I suppose she means you go slow. You want the thing watertight. She tells me that Mandarin has a simple grammatical structure. "Don't think too much," she says, and smiles. "Don't make it more complicated than it should be: subject, verb, object." She is a petite twenty-three-year-old, with shoulder-length, straight dark hair.

The gray living room couch arrived the week before, and we sit on it together. She has a quick smile and a great, high-pitched laugh. She wears red-framed eyeglasses and a purple sweatshirt with cartoon writing. I want to tell her that I often make things more complicated—that it's my nature. But now I'll try to follow her instructions. I'll try to build the boat.

It's important, here at the outset, to be realistic about Mandarin. Because Chinese is an old and vast lexicon, and there are thousands of those hand-drawn characters. And then the tones—four different intonations on rising and falling syllables. Things can get murky with the tones. You can say you'd like to go to the grocery store. Or at least that's what you think you said, but because you missed the fourth tone, you said something about a boyfriend in high school. This language is slippery.

Next Rose explains that you don't conjugate verbs for the future or the past. This seems fitting for a country in the middle of reinventing itself. She says English relies on logic and word sequences, but Mandarin is based more on graphics—the characters and nuanced meaning built up over hundreds of years. She teaches me the words for *weekend plans* and *elementary students*. She tells me how to ask a small boy his age. She says there are two little words I need to get a quick grasp of. Tiny words, really: *le* and *ge.*

*Le* is the word that turns the present tense into a memory. So if you went out and bought milk and eggs at the store, or if you got sick, you didn't really buy anything and you didn't really get sick until you insert *le.* Then you *have* gone shopping and you *have* become sick. And you can't buy apples at the market until you've learned to use *ge*—a miniature counting word. The Beijingren will look at you like you're speaking Russian until you insert the *ge: san ge ping gou* (three apples). A small detail—but I'm learning that the heart of this language, like most, lies here. If you have the patience, then you're back in the boat-building business.

It's slow going. There's the Chinese word *ma,* which takes a declarative and turns it into a question. *Ma* seems to carry the Mandarin interrogative on its back. Look at a simple sentence: "Tianqi hen re" (*The weather is very hot*). To flip a statement into a question, you put little *ma* on the end: "Tianqi hen re ma?" Then you're asking an actual question in actual Mandarin.

Rose is the Western name Wei Ling has given herself. So far in China I've met an Alice and a Sunlight, a Happy, a Flora, a Julia, a Margie, a Vanessa, and a Joy, and now three women named Rose. Rose is from the city of Guiyang in

Guizhou, one of China's poorest provinces. She's the only child of lower-middle-class parents who sound like they dote. They were able to pool money and send Rose to college in Beijing, quite a feat in this country, where often only the smartest and richest get to enroll. While she was in college, Rose met a boy who would like to marry her.

With Rose's help, I can now say "I want" in Chinese, and "I go." Putting the two verbs together has proved helpful: "Wo xiang qu" (*I want to go*). I use this combination in as many ways as humanly possible: I want to go to the *xue xiao* (boys' school). I want to go to the *chao shi* (supermarket). I want to go to the *yinhang* (bank). I want coffee. I want tea. I'm beginning to feel primitive. I tend to walk around Beijing making simple declaratives: "I want water." Or "I want to go home." There's an embarrassingly large amount of want on my end: I want, I want, I want.

Saturday comes—we've made it through another week and begun the day in prayer. Or at least the Blind Boys of Alabama have. I can't get enough of their beautiful voices. They're singing a song on the CD player about feasting on milk and honey: "All God's children gonna sit together one of these days, hallelujah." The Beijing sky plays tricks. It's a two-headed beast. Yesterday it was something to run from—thick and white and feverish. Today it's blue and warmed with a fat, autumnal sun that transforms the city into something that makes sense. A city at the center of the universe, where anything feels possible.

Thorne and Aidan eat their Honey Nut Cheerios and tap their feet to the music. Thorne is still singing more than usual, but it's tapering off. He lost one of his front teeth in the cafeteria yesterday, and his teacher threw it away by accident.

Last night Thorne and I co-wrote a note to the tooth fairy. It read, "Hello there. How are you? How was your flight? We are using a replacement tooth under the pillow (a tooth I lost back in July) due to extenuating circumstances. We hope you understand."

After breakfast, Tony and I drive with the boys and Lao Wu to a stretch of new art galleries inside a converted war munitions factory. The place is called Dashanzi. Or 798—the street address. There are hundreds of choices here: high art and low art and black-and-white photographs by teenagers who sell them from kiosks along the wide roads. The place hums with industry and grows so fast that no one can make an accurate map. The boys and Tony and I walk into the lobby of one big gallery, and there's a black sign announcing an Indian artist named Anish Kapoor. I can't tell where the exhibit is. Then over by the right side of the wall I see an open door to a tunnel.

Thorne pokes his head inside the tunnel, looks back at me once, then is gone. First I see him, then I don't. A wave of anxiety washes over me. Where is he? Down some long, winding labyrinth of performance art, and I'm supposed to go fetch him. I can tell there's a trick, that once I enter the tunnel I'm part of the exhibit. I want to go home. I can't get my bearings in Beijing.

Aidan says he needs to climb a huge, metal birdcage installed out on the street corner, and I wave Tony toward the door. "I'll go in," I say and poke my nose into the tunnel. "It's no problem."

I make it ten feet or so before the walls curl in on themselves like a snail shell, and I have to reach out and press my hands along the wooden sides. I can hear Thorne laughing up ahead. His voice echoes back amplified. I walk and walk and don't catch up to him. Anish Kapoor has shaped the tunnel in a way that forces you to turn in on yourself. You keep making tighter circles, but there's no sensation of getting closer to any ending, no light coming through from the other side. No sense of when there might be an arrival—seconds or minutes or hours. Inside the tunnel, I can see my fear of living in China up close. Fear of losing control, of being alone in this country, unable to manage for my kids. Fear of not being able to learn the language. Fear of not finding a way to belong.

This tunnel is cruel psychotherapy. I land at a circular patch of grass in the middle of a second white room. That's where Thorne stands, holding his hands in thick steam that rises from an opening in the ground. His face is rounder than Aidan's. Thorne is often quick to smile. He does not study life so much as eat it up—always looking for more. I get down on my knees and open my arms so he runs to me and I'm able to hold him like this for maybe five seconds. He seems at peace in the tunnel. At peace already in China. And could this be? Do my children already belong here more than I do?

Then he laughs and runs back through the darkness. Ten minutes later, I make it out alive. Thorne waits for me by the door. We walk toward Tony and Aidan in the birdcage and pass some heavy-metal Chinese teens. The boys wear low-rider jeans with wallets hooked to their back pockets on silver chains. They have long, carefully shaped sideburns and type text messages on their cell phones. A lot of the girls sport wispy bangs and orange-colored permanents. They are so hip they don't look like they belong in China—or not in the old China, anyway—but at least they have each other. That's the thing I'm coming to realize. How important it is not to feel alone in the tunnel—to know your people are waiting for you on the other side.

I stand next to Tony and can't begin to describe my anxiety back in the maze. It's already become a wordless thing. But what's left is this residue that somehow I'm the odd one out. Exposed. The one who can't give up her control. Tony riffs with the teenagers in Chinese, and they laugh and wear eager faces of people making that cultural connection—people crossing the language bridge. For a moment I feel language-less. Invisible. Like someone who isn't really here at all.

# I Don't Speak Chinese

It's time to wean the boys off the Lao Wu minivan school service. October is upon us, and Lao Wu was hired to drive Tony to meetings at Chinese banks, not to shuttle small children. The news is that Thorne's stopped singing—or at least the compulsive part of it has let up. He still breaks into song more than most six-year-olds, but not in that obsessive way that makes me uneasy. Right now he's doing some preemptive moaning in the hall about riding the bus. I push the down arrow on the elevator and hold the door with my arm. Thorne and Aidan step in, and though I'm only two feet away, Thorne begins to yell at me. "In case you didn't realize it, I don't speak Chinese!" This is true. "So how will we get help on the bus if we need it?"

Our move to Beijing has for me become a parenting lesson in how to parcel information: what not to tell, what to tell, and when to tell it. I'm trying to slow the information overload. I place my hands on each of their heads and gently push them along. Aidan stares at the sky and says out of nowhere, "China is a dream in my mind." I look up at the cement skyscrapers in Park Avenue. The sky is filmy white with smog and the buildings are the color of putty.

The boys have been intrepid until now. But the shadow of

the school bus has rattled them. "What will happen if we miss the bus?" Thorne asks. I say if we miss the bus, we take a taxi to school. But I've decided we can't miss the bus. Because in a taxi, we'll be relying on my Chinese, and I won't be able to say the school address in Mandarin.

There's a crowd at the bus stop: Chinese moms and house-keepers called *ayis* and all kinds of kids. I try to act like I know where to stand and which bus to look for. I think the boys can tell I'm faking. It's not that I'm trying to *fool* them; I'm just trying to incite confidence. I want my body language to inspire—to say *We're going to be fine in Beijing. We're going to like taking the bus. We're going to love living in China.*

"The bus will be fun," I tell the boys while they each hold on to one of my thighs. It must already be ninety degrees on this still, windless Monday. Eight o'clock comes and goes, and then an enormous coach bus covered with red and white Chinese characters pulls in. Thorne squeezes my leg tighter and begins to cry. I keep a hand on his arm while I talk him down. But I'm hot and flustered. For some reason I decide getting the boys on the bus is a referendum on our entire move to China.

I only have three minutes to convince them. The school handbook makes it clear: the bus waits the full three and then leaves. The rest of the kids have gotten on and everyone is waiting. I'm not above bribery. There's a Taiwanese-American boy named Eric who recognizes Thorne from first grade. Just before Eric climbs the last stair onto the bus, he turns and says, "Hey, Thorne, do you want to sit with me?"

What a gesture. What a random act of kindness from one six-year-old to another. I almost cry out of gratitude. Thorne cannot hear Eric because he's begun to hyperventilate. "Listen." I turn to Thorne and speak slowly and loudly. "You know there will be treats."

"Treats?" Aidan perks up. He's been standing behind Thorne's right shoulder, watching to see how things will play out.

"Yes, treats." I brush a tear off Thorne's cheek. His skin is smooth. He still sounds like he can't get enough air and I wonder why I'm not figuring out another way to get them to school. Why we've brought them to China in the first place. "You both get on this bus, and when you get home, I'll take you to Jenny Lou's."

"Jenny Lou's!" Aidan smiles and makes for the bus door. "Jenny Lou's has Starburst." Tony thinks I've already turned Aidan into a sugar addict in China. But when my husband harps, I remind him that now is not the time to get health-conscious on me. We're living in one of the world's most polluted cities, so could he please not get holier-than-thou about fruit-flavored candy.

Jenny Lou's is a store—Chinese-owned—that caters to foreigners. That means it carries a boatload of processed, artificially preserved foods from countries like Russia and Australia and France. There's pepperoni and sardines and Pepperidge Farm cookies and Marshmallow Fluff. There are egg bagels made by a Chinese American woman recently returned from Brooklyn. The food is wildly expensive, even though the store appears to be falling down, with mildewed ceilings and piles of dirt in the corners of the produce section.

I read the school guidelines carefully in June before we moved. They explained how convenient the bus service was: picking up and dropping off kids at the front gates of apartment buildings all over Beijing. I knew the city had the newest drivers in the world. So many cars run over pedestrians here that the government doesn't report the statistics. "I'm driving the boys to school in China," I told Tony last August in our kitchen after the kids had gone to bed. Right, Tony nodded, and kept making a list of vaccinations we needed for our visas.

"No buses," I repeated. "No buses driven by strangers on Beijing highways." Tony nodded again. What he didn't tell me was that I would have no choice.

Thorne doesn't care as much about sugar as Aidan. In the end, my promise is twofold: Starburst at Jenny Lou's, and thirty minutes of England's World Cup qualifier match on Rupert Murdoch's Star Sports channel. "Deal?" I say.

"Deal," Thorne mumbles. Then he climbs on and sits in the front seat and bends his head so he can't see me. The bus leaves and I walk back to the apartment feeling deflated. It's not the march of triumph I imagined. Instead, it's another one of those confused mother walks: walk of guilt with a little bit of victory mixed in. The Bad Mother chorus starts up in my head. I read in some parenting book that you're not supposed to bribe your children—you're not supposed to cave. I didn't cave, did I? I got them on the bus.

The sky looks smoggy. But this is an understatement, so let me try again. I can't write "thick, noxious fog" every time I want to invoke bad air, so I'll just call it smog, and you can imagine the worst. I walk toward the hutong, past the circular lawns of scrappy grass. It seems to be hard to make things grow in this city. The soil is thick clay. Another elm sapling has died outside our front door. The gardening is done by a full work unit of men in torn black blazers. The black blazer seems to be the uniform of the entire Beijing working class. I do not fully understand this. It's a polyester blend, and the majority of men do manual labor wearing the blazer and black loafers.

The gardeners work until six at night digging dirt holes and pruning and hauling out dead things. There's one woman, and she wears black jeans and a polka-dot blouse—no blazer. I've been told these gardeners used to have hutong houses where the Park Avenue apartment towers have been built. In

China there is a great deal of imbalanced quid pro quo: you let me tear down your house that's been in your family for five generations, and I'll give you a job for two dollars a day gardening in the multimillion-dollar apartment compound we build on your land.

At the pond, scores of men and women jump up and down in place. Under one tree, a small group of gray-haired men and women practices tai chi. Then, further down the path, other couples—men with women and women with other women—practice ballroom dancing. During the Cultural Revolution dancing was outlawed, along with other things. Birds, for example, were banished. Mao didn't like them. Now the dancers bow to one another with big smiles on their faces, as if they realize how lucky they are to be here, at the start of the next century, waltzing in Beijing after all China has lived through.

A clutch of older men walk to the field behind the pond carrying pigeon cages covered in blue flannel blankets. They hang the cages on the trees, then open the doors, and the birds fly over the sky in formation.

Last Saturday, my first Chinese friend in Beijing, Sabrina, came over with her kids, who go to school with Thorne and Aidan. Sabrina grew up in Beijing. She stood in my living room and looked at the hutong and said it had been housing for work units during the Cultural Revolution. The buildings are long and narrow and set in rows like army barracks, each made of gray concrete with a flat roof.

Sabrina explained how the revolution took the parents away. She was raised by elderly grandparents and was lucky to see her parents for visits. Then she pointed at two sets of common bathrooms that sit in front of the hutong, where people come and go with buckets of water. Sabrina's family had a house in the city, a "square lot," she called it. But no toilet.

So all her life she walked the alley to the bathroom. "That is why"—she smiled—"when you go into the hutong, you see people walking in bathrobes and slippers. They have just come from the toilets."

I've heard people say that the entire neighborhood out back will be razed after the Olympics. Right now the government has put a freeze on demolition inside the city. Hundreds of skyscrapers have to be ready by the opening day of the Olympics, August 8. The race to finish goes on around the clock. Sabrina told me the hutong out back won't be saved. "It is not pretty," she said, and so it will go.

Today, thirty blue flatbed trucks are parked in front of a string of one-story cement shops. Each shop is the size of a small woodshed and has a stone roof. A woman sits in a chair guarding one of the shops. People smoke and spit and stop their bikes and rickshaws to talk. Some eye the woman's concrete powder. Finally, two men in black blazers open a bag and sniff. Another woman in a blue sweat suit sweeps in front of her cement shop. The wind blows the dirt back toward her. Halfway down the block, a man puts out two small plastic tables and stools and cooks what looks like rice soup in a wok he's lit from a gas burner on the ground. A couple of men sit down to eat.

Someone would have noticed by now if the two new American boys hadn't gotten to school, right? A lot of this expatriation seems to be about trust in strangers. About faith in some larger, global force of good. Because my children are out on the Beijing highway without me. Maybe I shouldn't have been such a hard-ass about the bus. They're small children.

Drivers congregate around the flatbeds and stand in a circle and smoke. When they smoke, they also spit. Smoke and spit. Spit and smoke. This is the sequence. I'd heard about the spitting in China before we arrived. I'd even read about a government campaign to eradicate spitting before the Olympics. Apparently, some of the rich Chinese don't like the spitting. They write essays in international magazines about how the spitting will embarrass China at the games. One of the problems seems to be that people believe spitting is medicinal, that it clears the lungs. Most of the spitting I've seen involves a deep, honking sound that calls up any mucus rattling around. Then silver dollars of phlegm get left along the city sidewalks and streets like calling cards. It's impossible not to step in them.

The woman at the concrete shop has two real customers. She jumps up. The men reach into one of the bags and finger the concrete powder. Then they pull out cigarettes and light up. Once the smoking is done and the bargaining seems complete, they pile bags in the back of the cart they've pedaled to the shop.

A young woman pushes a rickshaw filled with green vegetables. She's come from the outdoor market, I bet. I walk down the alley to the market and fill a plastic bag with long Chinese beans. Then I grin at the teenage boy selling them and hand him a five-RMB note, and he smiles and gives me change.

I walk back to the apartment and sit at my desk and stare out my bedroom window. I've got my laptop plugged in and I begin an e-mail to my dear friend Sara, about the amazing number of people who come and go from the public toilets every few minutes. E-mail has become my best friend in China. It's how I talk to people back home. I've always had a love/hate thing with e-mail. I can still feel its tyranny—the way e-mail imposes a false sense of urgency, and how it replaced letter writing almost overnight. But for me the love now outweighs the hate. Because I can miss my mother and write her a note about the color of the China sky, and maybe

I'll hear back from her in two minutes if the timing's right. I can write to my great friend Winky, who lives two doors down from me in Portland, and tell her how much I'm thinking of her. Then she sends me a photo of my house with the October leaves piling up on the lawn.

When the boys return home on the bus, I stand on the sidewalk and wave them out. "How was it? How was the ride?" I ask, breathless. But I'm more worked up about the bus now than they are.

"So-so," Aidan says. Thorne dribbles a soccer ball on the concrete without answering. I have already called Lao Wu on his cell phone and he can take us to Jenny Lou's. We climb into the van. This is the victory drive for Aidan. At the store, he walks around the candy aisle three times before choosing.

After we buy the treats, we climb back in the van, and Thorne says, "There's a boy on the bus named Andrew from Shanghai who hit me."

"Hit you?" *Oh God.* "Hit you where?"

"Eric and I sang a song about Andrew and Molly getting married and so he hit me. On the shoulder."

"Did it hurt?"

"It's okay, Mom," Thorne says calmly. "We're friends now. After he hit me, Andrew gave me some of his Doritos."

We drive the rest of the way home in silence while I go over the day's sequence of events. The ending is still the same—the boys are safe. They eat their candy and stare out the van window. When we get back to the apartment, we turn on Star Sports and watch the soccer on the couch together, both boys' feet in my lap.

# Xiao Wang

October is also the month we hire a woman named Xiao Wang to be an ayi—the Chinese word for magical housekeeper. And how completely typical: the Americans go to China and create a small feudal system. It feels like that sometimes. The whole thing is unsettling and awe-inspiring: Xiao Wang will come to our apartment every day, and just for starters, she will clean the floors and iron shirts.

When I was growing up, it was a big deal when my mother hired Mrs. Endicott to come vacuum every two weeks. But many of the Chinese people I've met here seem accustomed to having staff—comfortable with domestic and professional hierarchies that for many Americans are unheard-of. Someone to cook your meals every day? Come on. Someone to iron your shirts? You've got to be kidding. Someone to help clean the bathrooms and organize the socks and load the dishwasher? You can't be serious.

The name Xiao Wang means "little Wang," and we got word from a friend of a friend at the boys' school that she was looking for work. I believe the other magical thing Xiao Wang will do is buy food to cook for our dinner. Xiao Wang comes to work on the first day wearing tight, acid-wash jeans and a bright pink, long-sleeved T-shirt with Chinese writing on it. She is a reed-thin thirty-year-old woman with shoulder-length black hair and pretty eyes, who doesn't speak English except for a few key words I'll come to rely heavily upon, like *yes* and *no* and *okay*. She has a two-year-old boy, a young husband, and a quick laugh, and will work for us from eleven in the morning until five in the afternoon.

Many Chinese people I meet here have multiple ayis—an ayi for each child, an ayi who cooks, a different ayi who cleans. There's a whole ayi industry in China. I interviewed four other women for Xiao Wang's job. The interviews were excruciating gatherings at our dining room table. The candidates were young Chinese women in their twenties who'd come straight from rural villages. I'm not sure they'd been in Beijing for more than an hour before the ayi agencies hired them.

The e-mail I got from the agency rep said, "Each candidate is proficient in English and knows how to raise children." It wasn't that I didn't find any of the women promising—they were each kind and hopeful in their own way. It was just too arbitrary to conduct a job fair in my apartment and choose one girl over the others. Each sat at the table and stared quietly at me and I stared back, trying to figure her out. Trying to get a feel.

But that was almost impossible. None of the girls spoke any English. They all looked nervous. Each had memorized a series of rote responses in English. I asked, "Have you ever taken care of children before?" All four of them smiled and said yes at the same time. "Do you like to cook?" Same response.

When I met Xiao Wang, I hired her on the spot. She laughed a lot and said in English that she really wanted the job. She needed the job. Then she made an unsolicited pledge to learn a new English word every day. I said I would do the same with Chinese.

. . .

In October, we don't see Tony much. He's busy with the new job. He stays up until the middle of the night talking to people in the States about the fact that the Chinese don't like to pay for projects until they're completely done. He's started having nightmares about how to say phrases like "risk management" and "credit allocation" in Mandarin. There are big, dark circles under his eyes. I've never seen him this stressed out before, or this exhilarated: he wonders if his employees enjoy his brand of leadership—a style I describe as calm and trusting. He's trying to build company pride and hosting monthly Friday after-work parties. He's hoping to get the new hires to bond. But it's harder than he thought it would be to open a business here. More challenging in every way.

His Chinese is my most valuable commodity here. I still feel as if I've been cast illiterate, or perhaps mute, in this country. I call Tony at work because the gas stove won't start and the water in the shower doesn't come out. Yesterday, I think I showed restraint by only dialing his office nine times.

"Two years," I say to the Chinese woman named Flora when she asks me at the playground how long we'll be here. Her daughter, Samantha, is in Thorne's class. I watch the three children climb up the metal slide backward and then I quickly look up to the sky. "Two years," I repeat to myself slowly. "We will be here two years."

Today is what people in Beijing call a "bad air day." It's a mild euphemism for when the sky becomes so foggy I can't see skyscrapers out my bedroom window. Right now we're inside a low-pressure system that's trapped clouds and moisture over the city like a lid. The smog begins to sting my eyes.

We'd heard there were throngs of expats here, but it turns out many of them have fled to the suburbs. Beijing is just too dirty, too loud and polluted, for some. I overheard a Belgian woman at the visa office yesterday say Beijing lacks charm. Lacks history. She's holed up in a French diplomatic compound outside the city. She'd lived in Shanghai the whole year before, she said. "Shanghai has flavor," she explained to her friend seriously. "It's so much better. But Beijing"—she shook her head—"no. I won't live here."

There are government initiatives to make the air better before the Olympics—they have a "blue sky" goal of 150 days in 2008. This seems like a high number. Each day you can check pollution levels on a government Web site, but I don't need to look at the ratings. It might be helpful to understand that the Clean Air Act in the United States limits healthy "fine particle pollution" concentrations to thirty-five micrograms per cubic meter. Levels between fifty-one and one hundred are moderate, and anything over a hundred is harmful to "sensitive groups," including children and the elderly. It's weird to live like this, but I've decided to make friends with the pollution. It's like a Down East fog rolled in from the outer banks. Soupy. Which is a word we say in Maine when the fog won't burn off.

Pollution here seems to have a lot to do with wind. The city sits at the northern edge of the North China Plain, bounded on the north and west by mountains. Wind blowing south or east pushes things out of the city. North or west winds leave things over the city, along the mountain front.

Tony likes to check the ratings. He calls me at the playground on my cell phone and asks if I want to know today's pollution numbers. "No," I say. "I don't want to hear it. I'm sure it's worse than I think."

He isn't listening. "One hundred fifty and rising," he says, as if I'm interested. As if I can't already tell it's bad by the headache I feel coming on, and the fact that I can't see the trees across the street.

"Thank you for that," I say. "I'm hanging up now. You've made my day."

That night, after the boys go to bed, Tony opens a bottle of wine and we sit on the couch so our legs are touching and look down over the Fourth Ring highway and farther out to the crowded skyline. It's Friday, and it feels like we haven't been alone together in weeks, because we haven't. I've missed him. Before we moved here I forgot to plan for his absences and all the work he'd have.

"How are we doing?" Tony asks and takes my hand in his and kisses it. He's a stealth romantic. We forget our wedding anniversary for years in a row. But, as we both like to say, our love is the key to the whole operation. And right now the operation is stationed in China, where Tony likes to keep a running score of our wins and losses. "Is China beating us this week?" he asks, and smiles.

"On Monday," I answer. "We won. Clearly we won because we had the good luck to hire Xiao Wang." I take a sip of wine and try to smile. "But today was different. Today it was too smoggy for the boys to play outside at recess."

Tony nods. "One for us. One for China."

Sunday morning comes, and the boys eat French toast at the dining table. Tony walks in from the hall and kisses them good-bye. He's flying to Shanghai for meetings all week. Right before he leaves he gives Thorne and Aidan a speech: "Be kind to each other and more important, be kind to your mother." I stand by the table and feel like our family is some throwback to the fifties. I'm the housewife whom the kids are badgered into being nice to? I'm more dependent on my husband than I've ever been.

I've learned that needing Tony and feeling close to him are not the same—need is about practicalities; intimacy is a mysterious underwater current. I bet Brie, the astrologer back in Maine, would attest to this difference. I wouldn't be surprised if Saturn wants me to cleave to Tony like some helpless bride and never give Neptune a chance.

Tony kisses me on the lips and he's gone. By 9:00 a.m. I've announced the second round of Monopoly—the special edition Red Sox version. Before the game even starts, Aidan comes out of his room wearing a full Brazilian soccer uniform: blue shorts and yellow shirt and knee socks, plus the shin guards. Aidan is a big costume guy. For one year in Maine he lived in a red and blue Spider-Man suit—wore it to school and the supermarket and the playground. He took the business very seriously. And after a few months, once I understood it, I did too. Because when Aidan was Spider-Man, he was bolder and braver and more himself in many ways than when he took it off. I could give him that. I could let him be Spider-Man as long as he wanted because hey, the world can be a scary place, and we get our strength wherever we can find it.

On Friday Aidan's teacher, Carmel, e-mailed to say that Aidan walked into the classroom that morning, took off his sweatshirt, and said, "I hate it here." Carmel is seeing this as a good thing. She's such a positive woman she's been able to convince me it's healthy that Aidan is communicating how he feels. Getting it out.

I think Thorne is who we have to pay attention to. Because he isn't saying much. Right now our camp leader is lying on the couch staring at the ceiling, when what he needs to be doing is organizing our day—out fixing the flagpole and then planning a scavenger hunt.

"Come roll the dice, Thorne," I say. "It's your turn."

Thorne doesn't have any real friends yet, and this is a painful thing for a mother. He used to have friends. Friend making was one of those seamless things for him. Now when I drop him off at school, he hangs around the teacher, watching the other boys play soccer. Diba has e-mailed me that Thorne is making strides. She says some of the kids are warming to him. *Warming to him?* And it's hard for me sometimes not to storm into the building and make friends *for* Thorne. Just go meet a few six-year-olds in the hall and say, *Hey, this is Thorne. He's fun. What's your name?*

"I hate school," Aidan says to me now. "And you know why, Mom?" He flops his whole thin body into my lap. "You really wanna know why?"

"Please tell me." It's my turn. I lean and move my man six spaces, to Yawkey Way.

"Because you can't wear tie-up shoes. You have to wear shoes without laces."

"You mean with Velcro?" I look down at him and try not to laugh. I've already learned about the Velcro problem. Carmel also told me on Friday that Aidan wasn't fast enough at tying his laces yet. She'd like us to get some sneakers with Velcro but I keep putting it off—hoping that maybe Aidan can increase his tying speed over the weekend. I don't want to have to go to a Beijing shoe store.

"Yeah, that's it. Velcro," he says, and begins to suck his thumb.

The trick with Aidan is to make him think you're on his side. He needs to know everyone is rooting for him. And we can never openly laugh at him—even if we're only laughing because what he says is funny. "So you hate the school because you have to wear shoes with Velcro?" I ask. He nods. "Then that's a problem." I rub his hair. "I bet that's really frustrating."

By that afternoon Lao Wu is driving us to the Lufthansa Shopping Mall for sneakers with Velcro. Aidan falls asleep in the minivan and wakes up quietly saying, "I wasn't planning on this. I wasn't."

"Oh, Aidey." I'm sweating. What I want to say is that I wasn't planning on this either.

"I knew I wouldn't like it here." Aidan is getting louder now. "I knew I wouldn't like China." Lao Wu parks the van in a spot outside the mall, and I pull Aidan onto my lap in the front seat. Then Thorne and Lao Wu get out and stand in the parking lot singing a Chinese folk song. But Thorne keeps waving for me to get a move on. I tell Aidan that China will get better. Easier. "Week by week we'll have more fun. Just you wait," I say. "Real fun." Aidan nods and wipes his nose with the back of his hand. At least I can still reason with him. I open the door, and we climb out of the passenger seat together.

It's probably true that a lot of my worries about the boys in China are the same worries I'd have in the United States. Mothering small children for me is a math lesson in worrying: what part to subtract? What part to pay attention to? It's a constant tally sheet. Some things just feel exaggerated here. I can't seem to make everything better in China. We've given ourselves up to the Greater Forces. Dropped into the river, and now we each have to swim for ourselves. I am counting on the boys to do that. I am counting on the fact that they can swim.

# Chabuduo

Xiao Wang and I reach a language stalemate. It's the first day of November, and I try to tell her that two maintenance men will be arriving to install a metal rod in Thorne's closet, so we can hang clothes in there. I think I explain in Chinese that a closet is a place to put clothes (*yifu*), but I'm not making sense to her. In the end, I motion for her to follow me, and we walk back to Thorne's room, where I open the door to the closet and say, "Closet. This is a closet." Then we both laugh.

When the maintenance men ring the doorbell, I stand in my wool socks in the hall and stare at their lips. Tony has arranged their visit over the telephone. The men speak to me in what I now call machine-gun Chinese, and I nod as if I have some notion of what they're saying. Then they take off their black loafers and walk into my apartment in their white socks like they own it. It's noon, and I whisper to myself that if these men are going to rob Xiao Wang and me and tie us up with ropes, they should get it over with. I don't know the Chinese words for getting help. Besides, I don't know anyone who would come for us anyway.

But the men are laughing with each other. They smell like nicotine. I leave them inside Thorne's closet and go into the kitchen to chop onions with Xiao Wang. She's teaching me how to use the cleaver after she saw me cut a green pepper with a steak knife yesterday. That was when she told me her mother died of cancer. Last year, when Xiao Wang's mother got sick, she and her husband took their baby and walked away from their jobs in Beijing to go to take care of the dying woman. This is the Chinese way, Xiao Wang explained. When someone is sick, there's no question. You leave everything.

After they buried her mother, Xiao Wang and her husband came back to Beijing with the baby and couldn't find jobs. Her husband is a driver, but no one has been hiring. She says there are no jobs in her old village and the young people have left. Only old people stay in the small towns. Her whole family—including her husband's parents, who live with them—survives on wages Xiao Wang makes at our house. They don't have the proper Beijing ID—the *hukou* (residency card) that allows them free school and a little health care. The card can cost thousands of U.S. dollars on the black market. Without the hukou, Xiao Wang is like an illegal alien in Beijing. The police can stop her on the street anytime and send her to jail or back to Shanxi Province.

Xiao Wang makes three hundred U.S. dollars a month and works six hours a day. At the bus stop yesterday Flora scoffed at how much I pay Xiao Wang and said it's way too much. Flora thinks it's scandalous. Her ayi works twice as many hours as Xiao Wang and gets paid half as much. I want to tell Flora that this kind of domestic hierarchy is not my way. I'd like to explain that I *like* Xiao Wang. She washes the floors and vacuums the rugs and folds the clothes and has done more ironing in the last three months than I've done in my life. She is the housewife I've never been. All of which makes me grateful and uncomfortable and convinced we should be paying her more.

I make a pile of onions on the cutting board. Xiao Wang

seems relatively pleased with my work. She nods and reaches for the wok, and then the doorbell rings again. The maintenance men are still chatting in Thorne's room. I haven't wanted to interrupt them. Who could this be now? I look through the glass peephole. There's a man in a green China Mail uniform.

It took a while, but by now we've all but forgotten that there was ever a time in our lives when we got regular mail, or that there are countries where people check their mailboxes every day. Because we don't get mail in China. Haven't yet. But this man seems to be asking me to open the door so he can give me the big box he's holding. I say, "Hao de. Hao de" (*Good. Good. Okay),* and reach for the doorknob.

I carry the box inside. My mother has sent a gigantic care package of kitchen sponges (I can't find any here) and maple syrup (liquid gold at Jenny Lou's) and two alarm clocks (missing from every department store I've cased here). There are also jelly beans and chocolate kisses and late Halloween cards for both boys saying she misses us so much she can't stand it: *When should I come?* she writes. *Because I'm coming and I can't wait much longer!*

On the packing slip she's written the tax-happy "Used office supplies" in the description box as a way to bypass Chinese customs officers. Getting packages is better than getting e-mail. E-mail can be a tease—it forges an intimacy that leaves me wanting more when it's over. I hold the jelly beans in my hands, and our life here doesn't feel as isolating—doesn't feel as remote.

The next morning there's snow on the ground. Maybe just an inch, but the streets and alleys around the hutong are slushy, and the tops of the stone roofs are dusted white. Beijing looks like a winter postcard of Maine. I put on a Dan Zanes CD to get the boys and me through breakfast. Tony has flown to a southern city called Shenzhen for meetings. Thorne finishes his Frosted Mini-Wheats and then stands up to dribble a basketball in the hall. I'm thinking things are going reasonably well for a school morning. No one's fretted about getting on the bus. No one's had a time-out for hitting his brother. I yell, "Five minutes before we leave!"

This is when Thorne says casually, "I'm ready to go back now."

I have no idea what he means. "Ready to go where?" I look up at him from the floor, where I'm tying my shoes.

"Ready to go home," he says. "Back to the USA."

*Good God,* I think. *Where did this come from?* And then my next thought is, *So am I*—I'm ready to go home too. Maybe all four of us are? But I need to stop. I need to reassure Thorne. And the fact is, we can go back soon—but not just now. Not when Tony has started this new job. Not this year. So I ask Thorne about swimming class and which backpack he can fit his bottle of Chinese iced green tea in. This is when he says things aren't going well at recess.

"How do you mean?" I ask.

"The boys say I can't play tag because I'm too fast."

"What if you tried not to win all the time?"

"But why would you do that?" He looks at me like I'm deranged. "Why would you ever try to lose?"

The rest of the week Thorne finds something to cry about every night before he goes to sleep. His teacher says everything Thorne is going through is within the parameters of relocation stress. Completely normal. Even the crying? Even the part where Thorne is mean and insulting to me? Because that's going on too. Diba says she sees it all the time with kids who relocate and that I have to be patient. More patient than I've ever been in my life.

But now that Thorne is unraveling every night, I am unable to find that patience. Or that small room I built in my mind. I want things to go well here for Thorne. Part of that desire is self-serving—when the days are smooth for my children, they're that much easier for me. And it's hard to see him struggle. Some of my frustration has to do with the fact that Tony is not here. I can't quite hold the pieces together.

On Friday morning, I get the boys on the bus after a fight and walk back to the apartment under a thick white sky. I sit at my desk and stare at my novel, which makes me miss Keith—my great Kentucky friend on whom I've based a main character. Keith loved to iron clothes and pore over the *National Enquirer* and before he died he once made a memorable birthday speech: *Susan, go get busy in the baby-making department because with Tony's dark coloring and your long neck you're gonna pop out some beautiful babies.*

At eleven o'clock, Rose comes for our second lesson and teaches me the Chinese phrase for "I think": "Wo juede." What happens next is kind of crazy. I learn that in Mandarin, "to think" and "to feel" are the same word sometimes. Interchangeable. I get two verbs for the price of one. I cannot tell you how much this pleases me. I can now think and feel in Chinese. I'm certain this one verb is going to light up the entire language for me. "Wo juede" is going to crack the whole thing open. It feels like a turning point, because now I will be able to make unfounded judgments. And isn't that what being a foreign visitor is about? Forming ridiculous opinions about the new culture? Now I will be able to make more friends. Now I will be able to fit in.

And it's true—the new verb does help. I can now say "Wo juede tianqi hen hao": *I think the weather is good*. And I can say,

"Wo juede ni jiantian hen lei": *I think you are tired today.* But then I begin to wonder about the other things I wish I could say in Chinese—more complex things about how hard it is to trust the government's air pollution rating system, and where to find fresh bread, and why the Cultural Revolution was allowed to happen. But I digress.

I'm always nervous when Rose arrives because I've never studied enough. Today she teaches me how to say "My two sons go to school" and "I am forty years old." Halfway through the lesson, there's euphoria. It only lasts for seconds—but in that brief time I grasp the intricate machinations of the language. Its fun shortcuts and slang. Rose smiles and lets out her high-pitched laugh and I feel I'm gaining.

But then she says I'm not pronouncing the words emphatically enough. This is the thing about Mandarin—you have to speak it like you own it. When you say you're hungry you're supposed to act like you've been sucker punched in the stomach. Some words are meant to be spoken so loudly you'd think everyone was in a nasty argument. I like to speak Chinese quietly. I'm embarrassed by the sounds coming out of my mouth.

Rose teaches me the word *chabuduo,* which means "more or less." I decide I'll throw it into as many Chinese conversations as I can. I'll be able to say I like the architecture of the Ming dynasty chabuduo, when I don't really have a clear picture of how the Ming differs from the Tang. Chabuduo helps, because nothing feels precise here—not the cost of apples or the traffic on the way to the boys' school or freedom of the press. It's situational and changing hourly. So I can say to the taxi driver that I'll be back in two hours chabuduo. What I'm really saying is I'm untrustworthy—that I'm not sure what I'm talking about. And here in Beijing both are true. Chabuduo.

# "How to Handle the Stress
of an International Move"

Just before Thanksgiving, I get an e-mail from a woman I sort of know from the boys' school inviting me to a "sweater party" at her house. "Well, what is this?" I say out loud. A sweater party? I'm supposed to get to Netti's apartment at ten o'clock on Tuesday morning. Netti lives in a new building in the center of town called Seasons Park, across the street from a megamall. The e-mail goes on to say that at the sweater party, a woman will examine samples of any sweaters I've brought from home. Then this woman will knit me more sweaters, just like the ones I've brought, in different colors and yarns. All for super cheap.

Netti is on the ball. She is, for example, the person in charge of the bake sale at the upcoming school Christmas bazaar. I'm not sure we'll attend the bazaar, though Netti's signed me up to bring a cherry pie. I have never made a cherry pie in my life. I'm realizing that even in China, I'm not always a joiner and that meeting other women can be exhausting.

But I cancel Chinese class with Rose on Tuesday and make my way to Seasons Park for two reasons: one, I'm curious about what happens at a sweater party, and two, I want more friends here. Making friends in Beijing has been harder than I thought. I don't seem to meet the right women—or rather, I hardly meet any women at all, and it can get lonely here.

So I go to Seasons Park—another high, shiny black skyscraper in a cluster of skyscrapers under construction, and rise to the seventeenth floor. I put my coat down in the front hall and learn that the Sweater Lady has canceled. No one knows why. Now eight women stand around in Netti's living room clutching plastic bags of sweaters. We are, as expats go here, very international (two Americans, two Australians, one South African, one Cambodian, and one Korean). I've made small talk with half these women before at school.

We sit down on the white sectional and smile at one another and work to find languages we can speak and subjects we can handle with our limited, pooled vocabulary. We tend to use a very punctuated English with some Chinese thrown in. Netti puts out store-bought cherry Danishes and a home-made pumpkin soup. I'm too old for this. Some of the women look disconcertingly young—like they may, God forbid, still be in their twenties. I decide we'll either talk about something interesting soon—say about school, or the Chinese government—or we'll head home. (And that is my secret hope.)

This is about the time Netti suggests we play video games. More specifically, she wants to plug in a video game system called Wii. Several of the women jump up, excited. They've never seen Wii but they're already thinking of buying it for their families. Netti gets out the equipment: handheld gadgets and cartridges and remote controls. There are interactive cooking games, and knights-in-armor-going-after-dragons games. There are soccer and Ping-Pong games and a garage rock band game.

She turns on her large plasma TV (every new apartment in Beijing seems to have at least two) and we stand and help move the glass coffee table. Then I sit on the couch and watch four of the women play a game of video tennis. They hold white remote controls and swing their arms like they're holding tennis rackets. The ball pings.

I keep thinking someone is going to laugh and turn off the TV and then maybe we'll talk about what's going in South Africa or Cambodia. (No, I am not holier-than-thou. I'll make do with some good gossip about the teachers at school or a great new restaurant near my apartment.) But these women are not near stopping.

My kids would go bananas over Wii. That's where my conflict lies. Because for me the games involve too much standing in front of the television—an overdose of what my boys have come to call "screen time." The South African woman hits a forehand. She's sweating and turns to say the game is a real workout. Then Netti tells me she likes Wii, "because it's something to do as a family." Her words bother me. There have to be better things to do in Beijing with my husband and kids than this. I stand and say I have to go. Then I take a taxi home and chew on the Wii party for a few days. It makes sense that there are so many electronic gadgets here. As a journalist here recently wrote, the fancy Beijing parks are designed for emperors and concubines, not for active seven-year-old Chinese kids with soccer balls. And the winters are long and cold. So what seems to happen in the tiny apartments is a whole lot of video gaming.

Today I'm heading out into the city again. There's a seminar at school for parents. It begins at 2:00 p.m. Maybe I'll meet a new friend. The subject for discussion is "How to Handle the Stress of an International Move for Your Family." I want to tell the school counselors that they offered this too late.

At the seminar, a Taiwanese woman named Sunny invites us to her house for dinner on Saturday night. Sunny is Aidan's friend Max's mom. She and her husband, Roger, live with their two boys in a large complex called Global Trade Mansion. Max doesn't speak any English yet. He has wild, dark hair and enormous eyes—he's the kind of boy you spot in a crowd and want to say hi to. The last time I took Aidan to school, Max ran over to us on the playground so he and Aidan could press their foreheads together until their noses almost touched. This is how they worked out saying hello.

On the way to the dinner in the van with Lao Wu, Tony tells me he's nervous about work. "We have a press conference on Monday," he says. "Financial reporters will be there to interview me in Chinese."

I lean over and rub his shoulder in the front seat. "It's going to be great," I say. "It's going to be so interesting."

"It's about two different ways of doing business," he says. "I'm trying to bring analytics to banks that until now have operated on intuition and big personalities."

"You mean hunches?"

"Yeah. They may do some analysis of the market, but then they discard it. They still say they have to trust their instincts instead of data."

When we get to the sixteenth floor, we ring the bell and Roger greets us holding slippers. We take off our shoes and put on the slippers, and then the boys run to Max's bedroom to play superheroes. Three other families from Taiwan are there for dinner. The men work at IBM together and have recently taken a trip to Japan, where they drank a lot of red wine.

"This will be a wine-tasting party," Roger explains. "Red wine and Taiwanese food." There are bottles of Cabernet and Pinot Noir on the table in the living room, along with an assortment of snacks I've never seen. "This," Roger says, pointing me to a plate of shaved meat, "is duck throat. And

this"—he picks up a small bowl—"is dried chicken tendon."
I take a sip of wine and make a mental picture of which bowls
of food on the table to avoid. Roger and Sunny are warm,
open people, and they understand that boys, at least our four,
will run wild. And that is what these boys do—they change
superhero costumes and switch who's chasing whom, and
they crash about.

Sunny pulls me toward the dining table. She used to be
on television in Taiwan and she wears beautiful, complicated
clothes—three layers of black shirts over a dark pair of jeans.
She has a round, lovely face and enormous eyes. She's put out
so many dishes. "Start with the chicken soup," she says. "I
made it this morning." It looks delicious. I ladle broth into my
bowl and out comes a large chicken claw. I try not to jump. I
don't know Sunny well enough to make a joke out of it. I look
at the soup and the chicken's whole head is now on the surface.
I'm staring down into the beak.

Sunny points me to tripe and then to what looks like duck's
feet. "We are eating well tonight," she says. "We are eating
the specialties." I listen to the other women talk in Mandarin
and try to sip my soup without letting my spoon touch the
chicken claw. I'm thinking about how in America we don't
often know where our meat comes from and how sometimes
that's easier and what a hypocrite I am.

It's late now. Long past the boys' bedtime. There's a mob-
ster shoot-out playing on a flat-screen in Sunny and Richard's
living room. The men sit silently, plates in laps, watching the
movie. Tony joins them on the couch and kids come and go.
I stand in the hallway, and each time I look over at the screen,
someone is getting shot or maimed. I would like to go turn
off the TV, and that's how I know it's time to leave the party.

Max and his brother seem immune. They glance at a man's
bleeding head on the screen, and then they start eating duck

throat near the snack table. Aidan is there too—laughing and drinking green tea. How is it that my boys seem more comfortable in China than I do? I don't know Sunny and Roger well enough to say I'm leaving because of the movie. Nor do I know them well enough to say how glad I am we've met. These new friendships have boundaries. We're feeling each other out. And now I can't find Thorne—where is he? Sunny and I say good-bye at the door and we hug, even though I'm pretty certain hugging is not the Chinese way. Tony slips back inside and finally locates Thorne over at the snack table chewing on a chicken tendon and liking it.

After the weekend, Xiao Wang arrives on Monday and tells me her son is sick again with a bad cold and is doing lots of coughing. The boy has been ill every week I can remember this year. He coughs so much that he throws up and then gets dehydrated. It's gotten so bad, they have to give him IVs at the local hospital. Xiao Wang says they try to stick the line in his hands, but when that doesn't work they try the boy's feet, and yesterday they had to put the needle in her son's head. The boy begins crying as soon as they drive up to the hospital on Xiao Wang's bike.

I go find the local Beijing guidebook and give Xiao Wang a list of public hospitals in the city. Some of them focus on pediatrics and sound like they might be free. I tell Xiao Wang to stop slicing ginger and call these places. I say in my bad Chinese that maybe her son needs more than the traditional Chinese medicine they offer at her hospital—more than compresses and fluids. I worry that the boy needs Western drugs. And will that even be enough?

Xiao Wang herself has a bad hip. Today she puts her hand on her right side and grimaces. It hurts. I ask her if she's been to the doctor and she says yes, to a Chinese doctor. After the X-ray, he put some cream on her hip and some heat but didn't give her any medicine. It sounds like a muscle pull. I know Xiao Wang is worried about cancer and thinks she's going to die suddenly like her mother. It's implicit in her worry. I ask her if she's ever been given ibuprofen. I find myself saying the word loudly to her, and then I spell it out, i-b-u-p-r-o-f-e-n.

I want to give her something to help her pain, but am I going against a lifetime of traditional Chinese medicine practice here? Undoing the benefit of countless herbal remedies? She shakes her head. No, she's never had any ibuprofen. I walk down the hall to my bathroom, where I grab a family-sized tub of Advil. I'm now the American drug pusher.

I hand Xiao Wang her first pill and pass her a glass of water. After she swallows, I panic. What if she is one of the rare people allergic to ibuprofen? What if she goes into toxic shock? I ask her if she feels okay and tell her to go sit down in the living room—that I'll check on her every ten minutes and see if the drug is working. She lies down on the couch and rests. But the first time I pop my head into the room, she sits straight up and says her hip seems much better. So good, she says in Chinese. *Hen hao.* She gets up and makes herself some tea and asks if she can have more of the medicine.

I wonder what kind of cultural interference I've run. I get a Ziploc bag and fill it with red capsules, then tell her to go home and check on her son. I feel uneasy about the ibuprofen. I say in my rudimentary Chinese, "Please don't come to work if your son is really sick tomorrow. And wait six hours before you take another one of the pills." She nods at me, gives me a quick smile, and is out the door.

# Mongolian Hot Pot

Beijing's gone crazy for hot pot. There are hundreds of these places in the city—Mongolian-style restaurants with round wells in the tables for pots of boiling broth. Rose calls and tells me to meet her at her favorite, a low-slung place with red couches and dark paintings of Mongols on horses. We sit in a red wooden room that looks back to the street. Rose orders thin strips of beef and chopped chicken, handfuls of shitake mushrooms, tofu squares, piles of Chinese spinach and mustard greens. This is going to be delicious. And even though I pay her for these lessons, I'm calling her a friend. Sometimes she is the only adult I talk to all day.

The idea with hot pot is to let the broth come to a boil so the seasonings mature, then start with the beef, which is slowest to cook. Next you add the chicken and the tofu, followed by the mushrooms, and then at the end, the greens. When the beef is ready, Rose takes a strip that's floating on top, dips it in a dish of sesame sauce, and pops it in her mouth. Then she asks me whether or not I'm a Christian. She swallows half the word so it comes out "isjen." "Are you a isjen?"

I'm surprised and poke one chopstick at a piece of tofu. So far no one in China has talked to me about religion. I've been waiting for this chance. I have questions I want to ask. Can you even talk about God in China? And did the Chinese really abdicate faith when the Communists took over, or just bury it? But all I can think to say in the moment is, "Are you?"

Rose finishes chewing and announces, "The Chinese don't believe in God. We believe in ourselves. We believe in our things." I can't tell how far we're going to go with this talk. Mao, after all, banned religion, and now the whole subject, like so many here, seems dangerous. I know that unless you're registered with one of the Communist Party–sanctioned congregations, going to church here is still illegal.

"So do you believe in an afterlife?" I ask Rose. "Something after all of this?" I point to the rickshaws and bikes passing by the window.

"The Chinese believe in ourselves," Rose repeats. "We believe in our families and our jobs."

I'm thinking of that monk we saw in September on top of the mountain and how he chanted for hours inside the temple. I wonder what he believes in. Outside the restaurant, three migrant workers walk by carrying striped plastic bags full of clothes. They wear yellow hard hats, and their pants are dirty, as if they've just left the construction site. Each man carries a saw in his free hand. I wonder what they would make of Rose's statement: *we believe in our things.*

Rose puts the mustard greens into the hot pot and says she's only technically allowed to live in Beijing two more years, until her hukou expires. After that she'll have to get married to a Beijingren if she wants to stay. Her boyfriend is a complaint manager at a Beijing real estate complex who listens to people tell him what's wrong with their plumbing and heating. From what I can gather, most apartments in Beijing were built with shoddy materials, and there's a lot wrong with them, so her boyfriend is busy.

I ask Rose if she wants to marry him, and if she misses him

when she's not with him. "He is too fat," she says in English, and smiles. "I don't miss him." He calls her many times a day. Her choice is a common one—to marry the first boyfriend or not. But Rose's mother did not have these choices: to move to Beijing for college, to stay in the city and begin teaching Americans, to go steady with a boyfriend of her own choosing. And Rose has men to choose from. Because after decades of a one-child-only policy and a sharp preference for boys, China is experiencing a shortage of girls.

"I love American television," Rose says to me then. I think she's trying to change the subject. She never likes to talk about herself for long. "There is a show called *Prison Break*. Do you know it?"

"No," I say. "But I don't watch a lot of television." When I'm with Rose, she laughs so often, she makes me smile. In many ways, Rose is all lightness. She doesn't dwell on the past, and this, too, has been a surprise.

"In China we are obsessed with *Prison Break*. The lead actor, I am forgetting his name." Rose laughs again. "He is very handsome. And tall. He is someone I would not have to think about marrying. He has money. I would marry him right away. If you have money in China, you can buy anything."

"Even kids?" I ask, and she nods.

What the really rich do now, she says, is buy fake passports from Canada or Britain or some other Western country. "In 1976, the one-child policy went into effect. Many rich Chinese left China. They fled the country so they could have as many babies as they wanted on the new passports." She dips her chopsticks into the broth and brings up a piece of tofu. "Minority groups in China can also have more than one child, but the norm is still one-child families."

My eyes are wide while I listen to her. "You yisi," I keep saying over and over. "You yisi"—*that's very interesting.* Last week I took the boys to the hospital for vaccines, and outside the radiology clinic there was a picture of a newborn baby on a poster with words in English and Chinese below: "Girl or Boy. Let It Be." After so many home abortions and orphanage drop-offs, there's a boy windfall here. Villages of unmarried men.

Rose says, "I've heard the government might be relaxing the one-child policy. Soon if an only child from one family marries an only child from another, that couple will be allowed to have two children. And," she adds, "if you have an advanced degree from college, none of these rules apply."

"What do you mean, they don't apply?"

"If you have a PhD or some other kinds of master's degrees, the government lets you have more kids."

"What kind of degrees do you have to have?" I can't believe what she's telling me.

She says it comes down to money in China. "You have to pay big money for your graduate degrees here, Susan. And the degree gives you a certain status."

"This is not Communism, is it? This buying of babies?"

Rose dodges my question. "It's changing fast," she says. "So fast we can't keep up with it."


On Friday morning the boys go to school. I clear the breakfast dishes and load the dishwasher. Then I work at my desk until Xiao Wang comes. I meet her in the hall and ask how her son is. No more IVs, she explains in Mandarin, though he still has a bad cough. She also says her hip doesn't hurt as much and smiles and tries to hand me back the remaining ibuprofen. "Bu yao," I say. "Bu yao," and I put my hand over hers. *I don't want them back.*

Then Tony calls from his office—he wants to play hooky at

a sports bar and watch the New England Patriots on TV. I say I'll meet him. The Goose 'n' Duck Pub is on the first floor of a giant new complex called Green Lake just across from us on the Fourth Ring Road. Inside the pub, the lights are dimmed and the windows are frosted so it feels like midnight. It's a big place, with five pool tables and as many giant flat-screens. The wall behind the long bar is covered in colorful banners: NFL, NHL, NASCAR, and NBA. There are seven customers when we arrive. Five of them are Chinese prostitutes. They look like teenage girls who haven't been to bed since the night before. They wear smudged black eye makeup and tight nylon dresses. One of the girls has passed out with her head sideways on the wooden bar. Three others hold pints of beer in their hands and shimmy to David Bowie on the sound system.

The oldest-looking woman in the group plays pool with a foreign man in a rumpled tie and a blue Oxford. I take him for American. Somebody's father. Somebody's husband. There is one other customer in the place—a tall black man with a curly beard wearing a knitted skullcap. He nurses a Coke and taps his hands on the bar while he watches a Thai boxing match.

The waitresses wear denim overall-shorts. One of them takes Tony and me to a table near the bar. We sit down, and before I can mouth the words *Let's get out of here*, the back door to the bar bursts open. Three men pull a large Christmas tree behind them. The Chinese start holiday decorating early. I look over at the girl with her head on the bar. She might be fifteen. She hasn't moved. No one is paying her any attention. The pool game stops, and the man in the tie makes his way to the bar for his drink. He puts his arms around each girl and dances with them in a circle for a minute. It's now eleven thirty in the morning. The girls cheer him when he orders another round of shots.

I try not to stare. But it's hard. I point the blue Oxford out to Tony. "How often," I ask, "do you think men who work for you end up in bars like this with girls like that?" We're now having an argument at the Goose 'n' Duck Pub while the New England Patriots fall behind on the television screen.

"Never," he says. "I've never come near a bar like this with the people I work with."

"But just know," I go on, "if you ever call to say you're staying late to play pool with the guys, this is the scene I'll imagine: that man over there sinking the eight-ball while the girls in minidresses clap."

"You're unfair," Tony says. "No one who works for me goes to bars with prostitutes."

"But how can you be sure?" It was a bad idea to come. "And we've only just moved here," I remind him. "Who knows what will happen?" Three teenage delivery boys arrive with takeout: cartons of noodles and fried rice that they place on the bar counter for the girls.

They're hungry—except for the one who's still asleep with her head on the bar. They all sit down at the bar with the blue Oxford and dig in, shoveling the food gently into their mouths. I can remember that hunger after you've stayed up all night drinking. It was something my roommate and I did in college a few times. You get to a point where you're not drunk anymore. Dawn comes and you're starving and, in my case, regretful. Tony steps outside the back door of the bar to take a business call and leaves me alone. The waitress hovers until I order something on the menu called a lemon juice. She brings me a glass of margarita mix without tequila.

The girls finish eating, and the New England Patriots pull ahead in the fourth quarter. I want to get out of this place. Tony comes back, and I'm not sure if we're speaking to each other. We pay the bill, and on our way out, we see the blue Oxford moving to rack one more game of pool. None of the girls around him seems sure where things are going to go next. All of them are waiting for a sign.

On Saturday morning I leave the boys making paper airplanes with Tony in the living room and walk to the new French market called April Gourmet that's just opened in Tower Four of Park Avenue. A Dutch woman I know named Anke is there, browsing the three small aisles. She moved here with her two girls and her husband back in August when we did, and I met her on the playground. I smile and wave and then go stand at the meat counter and ask for salami. It's from Italy, and this is no small development for Aidan. Salami in China. He loves salami.

Anke moves in line behind me. "How are you?" I ask. She looks so thin that I can tell she's in trouble. The girl behind the counter hands me my slices, and then I ask for two inches of provolone.

"My husband is having an affair," Anke says, and smiles broadly. "I have three days to decide whether to leave him or not." Then she laughs. "I'm calling it Project Beijing."

"Wow," I say. I do not smile. I know smiling is not the thing to do right now. But I'm at a loss in front of the cold cuts. I make a concerned face.

"I am supposed to go to my husband's parents' place in Texas for Christmas," she says. "I can't go, can I? I've found photos of the woman and their secret e-mails. She's waiting for him, right now, in Malaysia."

I stand and stare at Anke and recall that her husband is an American engineer. "Well," I say and glance at my slices of cheese on the white counter. "Well." The problem is, I don't know Anke. There was a time when I wanted to. All fall, really, when I was trolling for friends. But Anke has always seemed distracted. I have a feeling that today Anke could use more than a three-minute talk about her marriage in the April Gourmet deli line. "Christmas can bring out the worst in people," I finally offer and then can't believe how trite I sound.

"I'll snap, won't I?" she says and looks away. "If I go to Texas, I'll snap?"

"Probably," I answer and look her in the eye. She seems jumpy. Unstable. She keeps looking around and smiling.

"Isn't this a great store?" she says quickly. "Today I've bought arugula and these nice tomatoes." She holds up her plastic basket for me. "But if I don't go with him," she says, "and I let him take the kids to the States without me, the lawyer I just talked to said I might never see my kids again. That he could keep my kids in Texas with his parents forever."

"Where's your own family?" I ask and turn to fully face her. "Where can you go with your kids and get away from him?"

"I'm a nomad," she says. "We just move around. Tom's job moves us around. I go wherever he goes. My mom lives in Amsterdam."

"Can you go to your mom?" I ask. "You should go to your mom."

"I think Tom's abusive," Anke says then. "Mean to the kids and always yelling at me. You know, I suspected him all fall. He kept telling me I was imagining it."

Anke has a five-year-old girl named Anna and a two-year-old girl whose name I don't know. I've got my cheese now and I step out of line. "Please call me. I can help if you need it. If he gets abusive. Really. Call me."

"I will," Anke says, and she seems happier now. I wonder if she's on tranquilizers. I would be if I thought Tony was going to leave me alone in Beijing with two kids for a woman he'd taken up with in Kuala Lumpur.

The last thing Anke tells me is about a place she knows in Beijing where you can get a great martini. It's right above the best foot massage place in town. "You've got to go," she says and hugs me. "The very best drinks." Then she smiles that smile. "I have three days to figure out what the hell I'm going to do."

"Call me if you need me," I say again and meet her eyes, then I walk to the counter with my basket of lunch meats.

When I get back to the apartment, Aidan and Thorne have set the table with bowls and Tony has made a broccoli soup. We eat together in the dining room and I eye Tony over my bowl. So much of our time in China so far has been about laying grounding wire—figuring out how to buy apples and salt. Learning how to pronounce Chinese verbs. I'm not sure how I would describe our marriage. It's certainly a partnership, but there are long stretches here where it doesn't feel romantic. Instead it feels like we're running a small overnight camp for American boys in Beijing.

*And what am I really doing here?* I want to ask Tony. *He* is out slaying corporate dragons, hiring a staff and meeting with the heads of some of the world's largest banks. I am trying to write every day, but it's hard to get my mind to settle. Maybe the astrologer was right. Because it feels like Saturn may be casting a long shadow. I've been avoiding my desk. I once taught an adult writing workshop in Boston. The informal title of the class was "Ass in Chair." No one in the group had written in years. I kept finding myself explaining that there's never any writing—not one word—unless the ass is firmly in the chair.

I take a sip of Tony's soup and remember to thank him for it. He's a kind man. He's made us lunch. Never before has our marriage felt more lopsided. In some ways Tony and I seem to be in a new marriage. The old one was changed when we got on the plane to come to China. We're both learning more here than we imagined. Needing Tony so much makes me resent him sometimes. There's a lot we don't say because the words would be redundant. We're almost each other's only friend here. Or at least he is mine. How at this exact moment I would gladly trade him for any number of women friends. Tony makes good paper airplanes and stands with Aidan now showing him how to fly them. The kids run down the hall to Aidan's room to kick soccer balls. I tell Tony about Anke and the woman in Kuala Lumpur. Tony doesn't lean back into his chair and say, *Don't leave anything out.* It's not that he wants to avoid talking. He just doesn't share my need to unravel the day's events through a series of sentences.

I could get frustrated with this. I take another sip of soup and wonder whether or not to point out his deficiency again. I put my spoon down and say, "I wish sometimes we had time to check in with one another. You know—a few spare moments to talk."

"We do have time. Right now. But you're talking about walking on the beach." The line comes from a fight we had five summers ago. We'd landed the rare Saturday babysitter and jumped in the car, but were too tired to go anywhere. Instead we parked by the side of the road in Phippsburg and fought over what we should do: go to a movie or take a walk on the beach. I wanted to be the couple that went for the beach walk and had interesting things to say. I wanted, in some unspoken way, to go back for a few hours to a time when we didn't have children. When we weren't so damned tired all the time.

So I sat in the car by the side of the road and said, "Maybe there are other things you'd rather be doing than walking on the beach with me." Then for good measure I added, "Take me home. I don't want to go anywhere with you ever."

It turns out that when you have babies, sleep deprivation

can be a dangerous thing. "So this is great," Tony said while I sulked in the passenger seat. "All this time we've been talking about walking on the beach, when we could have been walking on the beach."

I look at my husband across the dining table and tell myself that marriage is a continuum. We've taken ours on the road. I stand up and announce that I'm walking the boys to the playground. I want to give Tony a break. He's made lunch, after all. When I come back, he's written a note by the phone: *A woman named Anke called.* But there's no phone number. Tony tells me she said she'd call back. I haven't heard from Anke since.

# Piaoliang

The site for the Olympic beach volleyball sits in the park across the street from our apartment, and on a warmish December Sunday we decide to put on our parkas and investigate. Chaoyang Park is huge, with miles of picnic spots and paddleboats and enclosed basketball courts. We walk over to the ticket kiosk and stand in line to board one of a yellow fleet of golf carts.

The tour driver is yet another no-nonsense Chinese mother who half plays nice and tells us about the dilapidated amusement park rides we pass, and half chastises me for not having my children sit properly in their seats. One moment this woman wants to touch Aidan's hair, and keeps saying how beautiful he is. The next moment she's trying to scam Tony for another hundred RMB. She and her copilot wear thick blue park-issued polyester parkas, with small wool caps.

When we get to the stadium, our driver says in English that come August this place will seat ten thousand people. I look at the barren park and the piles of dirt and bricks left in the makeshift lot and wonder if the Chinese government will forgive us all if we stay home and watch the games on TV.

Outside the stadium is the biggest digital photograph of a volleyball player I've ever seen, and I haven't seen many. But this one must be ten stories high. The woman is diving for the ball in the sand, and her cleavage has begun to spill over. The golf cart stops here, and we look up at the woman: Aidan and Thorne and Tony and me, plus our pilot and copilot in their parkas.

The volleyball player has her arms outstretched to return serve, and the photo almost makes me blush. Isn't beach volleyball an American sport? The bikini and the woman wearing it and even the stadium itself hit a Chinese cultural flat note. None of these things seems to me like it belongs in China. Beach volleyball involves lots of bright, clear sunshine, tanning oil, an ocean breeze, and copious amounts of sand. Our driver makes a whistling sound between her teeth and puts the engine in reverse. Then she yells loudly at Aidan and Thorne in Chinese to turn around and sit up. They are officially scared of her now. That's when she reaches out to touch one of Aidan's plump cheeks. "Piaoliang," she says to Tony. *He is beautiful.*

Thorne has a friend at school named Molly, who is also beautiful. The tide has turned and Thorne now has several friends, Jiho from Korea, Mads from Denmark, Ted from China. This is sweet relief. It turns out that being fast at tag can also be an asset if you're placed on the right team. Molly is a thoughtful six-year-old Chinese girl with long pigtails and round wire-rimmed glasses. She likes to read and sing, and she and Thorne sit at their homeroom table together every day and talk for hushed minutes with each other about how neat their penmanship is and how many minutes they can hula hoop. Molly holds the playground record.

When you meet Molly you know right away that she's one of those wise children who understands more than her years.

Her brothers, Finn and Jack, are British boys with swatches of blond hair who love soccer and electric guitars. Their mom is the school principal—an incredibly talented blond Brit named Julie.

For months Thorne has talked about Molly at home, just a line or two: "Molly had a fall on the playground today." Or, "Molly broke her pencil this afternoon." Then he came home yesterday, found me in the kitchen, and said, "You won't believe this."

"Try me." I put my tea down on the counter.

"Molly's adopted!!! She told me today she's adopted."

"So interesting," I say, trying not to let my surprise show because I can't believe it hasn't occurred to him before. He's almost beside himself with excitement.

"The real mommy put Molly in a cardboard box and someone found her and took her to an orphanage."

Lately, Molly has decided that she feels like sharing her story with her first-grade class. Thorne still can't get over it. "Her real parents didn't want her. They put her in the box. But then Richard and Julie found her and they are her parents now."

We talk about adoption through dinner and how the new mommy and daddy love the babies they adopt just as much as the real mommy and daddy did. Aidan listens silently while he eats his dumplings, and then he tells me he would not like to be adopted. I nod at him. Next he pauses in his chewing, looks me in the eye, and goes one step further by announcing, "I've decided not to leave. I've decided now to stay in this family."

"Good," I say and reach for another dumpling. "Wise decision."

# The Bag Lady

One of the things you do when you're dating new women in Beijing is you go on a series of follow-up dates. It's very Jane Austen at first. I try to pay attention to the rules of etiquette: it often starts with an e-mail—maybe from a woman I sat next to at a school luncheon, for example. I'm supposed to reply to the e-mail and suggest a follow-up activity: a trip to the Silk Market to buy fake pashminas, or a hutong walk. Once we've begun the courtship, it's understood that it will play out for weeks, if not months—a carefully calibrated series of overtures. The only thing many of us have in common is that we live in China, and our children may go to the same school. So it's not unusual during these rituals for me to have pangs of longing for my friends back home and to consider throwing in the towel. I've also learned that "dating" takes up an inordinate amount of time.

But I invited Sabrina and her kids over for dinner last Friday, and now she's called to ask if I want to go handbag shopping with her. I think this qualifies as a follow-up date. Sabrina and I may be courting. I say yes to the handbag shopping for the same reason I said yes to the sweater party. I'm still lonely, and part of me knows that having friends in Beijing is a good thing.

I've been told by an Australian woman at the boys' school that if I ever need handbags, I should go to the Bag Lady. Her operation moves around every few months to outrun officials, so while Lao Wu is driving toward downtown, I hand Sabrina the Bag Lady's phone number on a piece of paper and ask her to call. Sabrina's father is one of the coaches of China's soccer team. She's spent almost her entire life in this city and knows the back streets. It will be easier if she gets the directions in Chinese. But the Bag Lady answers and wants to know how Sabrina got the number, because she doesn't like to sell to Chinese women, only to (gullible?) foreigners. She tells Sabrina the address, but warns her not to share it.

We head to an apartment plaza called Soho near the boys' school and take an elevator to the eleventh floor of Tower Four, then turn right and knock twice on the door at the end of the hall. There's a small glass window in the door, and after we knock, someone opens a curtain inside and stares at us. Then I hear a dead bolt pulled back, and a stern teenage boy looks us over, then motions us in.

It's the penny candy store of illegal purses—they're piled on tables and in boxes and along wooden shelves. The majority of them look the same: shiny and black, with one or two leather shoulder straps, and a brand name stamped in silver or gold lettering. There's the Prada section and then Louis Vuitton. There's Chloé and Burberry and Miu Miu, and over there are Givenchy and Ferragamo. While I take in the room, the teenage sentry turns and locks the door so we're caged in.

I can't help but think of what will happen if there's a police raid or a fire. I have a feeling the Bag Lady (which one of the saleswomen is she?) would keep us locked up for a long time if it meant outwitting the customs officials. But who am I kidding? If the officials wanted the Bag Lady shut down, they could have done it years ago. She and the police prosper in the spirit of corruption. Because I can tell by the stitching and the uneven brass hardware that the bags are fake. I can tell by the way the leather crinkles and by the smell of synthetic.

Before I got to China, several people told me the shopping in Beijing "would be amazing." But this has not been my experience. Instead, I've seen a lot of pirated merchandise meant to fit petite thirteen-year-old Chinese girls. At five feet nine, I am an Amazon here. Nothing fits. But the words "amazing" and "shopping" are still enough to entice me. They sound transformative. Like something I can't miss.

Sabrina and I stand in the crowded room and spend an hour picking up purses and hanging them off our shoulders. The saleswomen wait behind a long, low wooden counter for us to bring the bags to them to price. Tense and edgy, these women never smile. There are other expats with us—Italian and British women, and a trio from Australia. They try on bags and bring them to the counter to haggle. The bags are expensive for the black market. One of the shiny black Pradas will cost you $200 U.S. The silver Tod's, $175.

I once had a student in Cambridge who wrote that she loved shopping because each time she went into a new store, she got a chance to reinvent herself. I'm not sure who I've become at the Bag Lady's—I appear to be an expat American riffling through the Gucci clutches hoping to find one that looks real enough to carry at my cousin Reagan's wedding next summer. I appear to care. But I'm posing. Before I moved here I thought only Americans had religious conversions in the church of consumption, but China has the fever too. Maybe more so because of the catching up they have to do.

Fake bags conjure up the bad things I've heard about the black market: child labor, sweatshops, slashed wages, illegal border crossings. Millions of people in China are supported by the black market—from fabric middlemen to seamstresses to drivers and retail clerks. What this says about a country's economic future is unclear. I've read reports that corruption is so rampant in China, it alone will bring down the government.

Sabrina and I walk away without a bag. For me there's relief. Once we get back down to the pavement, I breathe easier. I didn't like being locked up in a room with hot merchandise. Sabrina is disappointed. She was hoping for a Louis Vuitton in snakeskin, and they didn't have it. I have yet to see her pay full price for anything. She tries to bargain over the cost of our dumplings later at lunch when the waitress brings the bill. Before we say good-bye outside the restaurant, she tells me that next week she's going to take me to a better bag place. *An even bigger secret.* But I can't mention it to anyone. She's sworn me to secrecy. It's in a food market behind the new American embassy, and the bags *only come out at night* after the police have gone home for dinner.

During our dinner that night Thorne says Aidan is going to marry a Korean girl in first grade. At Thorne's seventh birthday party last November, one of Mi-cha's braids unraveled while she played kick the can. Then she and Molly ran over to me and asked me to fix Mi-cha's hair. Both little girls stood stock-still with serious faces while I began to rebraid. I was so glad I remembered how.

"You're going to get sexy with Mi-cha," Thorne teases Aidan. Tony listens, and I raise my eyes at him and remind Thorne that Aidan isn't getting sexy with anyone. "I won't marry Molly," Thorne adds. "Until I am at least twenty-five. But Aidan's going to get sexy with Mi-cha."

How is it Thorne knows the word *sexy*, and how can I make him stop using it? Aidan got off the bus last month and announced he'd learned a new naughty word, *fook*. A fifth grader named Brandon taught it to him. It took me a while to realize what he was trying to say.

But *sexy* is new. "Guys," Tony says casually while he takes a drink of water, "what's this new word you're saying?"

"Rashid taught it to us today," Thorne chirps. "Ali and Rashid." Ali is in Thorne's first-grade class, and Rashid is his older brother. Their whole family went home to Bahrain for the winter holidays. Before they left, their mother came into first grade wearing her head scarf and explained the Muslim fasting tradition of Ramadan. I went in to the class the week after and showed the kids how we decorate Christmas trees in America and put presents underneath. I felt sacrilegious.

"Sexy is not something you get with other people," Tony explains to the boys. "It's a way some people like to be. Or dress." Then Tony is silent.

I'm at a loss. Where does our talk go from here? "It's a grown-up word," I add, but I sound too mysterious.

"Like Amos," Aidan adds.

"Like who?" I ask.

"Amos. You know. Like calling someone an Amos," Thorne explains. "The place in your bottom where the poop comes out."

"Rashid said it was where you poop," Aidan says seriously.

Tony coughs into his water glass and I can tell he's having a hard time trying to not lose it. "Oh," I say and swallow a laugh. "Let's not say that one either. No Amos and no getting sexy."

# How Long Have You Lived Here?

Two uniformed police officers stopped me outside Tower Five today and asked if I had my registration papers and passport. I'm so used to the faux-military look here that at first I thought the officers were security guards. One of them carried a clipboard. Then I saw the word "Police" stitched in black thread on their white shirts, and my heart began to beat faster. For many reasons, it seems better to avoid the Chinese police while in China. The best one I can think of this week is reports of villagers who come to Beijing to protest the demolition of their family houses. They make it to the police station, where they're placed in what the foreign press calls "black jails." "Black" because the detainees have no charges against them and no sense of when they might get released. The whole operation is unofficial but sanctioned, just like the black market.

I told the officers my husband had taken the passports to the Chinese visa office to get the new, long-term work permit, and could I possibly call my husband to see where the paperwork was? Both officers listened intently and then followed me inside the lobby. I got nervous then. I had no idea where the passports were. Tony had taken them a week ago. The law in China is that you're meant to carry your passport with you at all times. The passports are gold. But no one moves around with them in Beijing. The chances of losing the passports on the streets are too high.

"How long have you lived here?" the woman officer asked me while we waited for the elevator. She was not friendly. She was a vehicle of the state with clear operating instructions, and I was sweating. If the officers followed me up to the apartment there would be a problem. A sinking feeling overcame me then. How do I say this? I felt culpable for sins. Guilty of many trespasses against the Chinese state. Hadn't I written scathing e-mails to friends about the way you aren't allowed to speak about the Tiananmen Square massacre here? I'm sure the police would read those once we were inside the apartment. And sophomoric rants on the cult of Mao and the collective Chinese amnesia? The officers would read those too, and then what would they do with me? I knew the policing operation was unpredictable. Sometimes foreigners got brought in—mostly Western journalists—for being in the wrong place with the wrong officer in a bad mood.

"I have lived here four months," I said slowly and tried to make my face look relaxed.

"Four months?" the woman officer repeated and cocked her head at me.

"Four." I cringed—four is the unluckiest of Chinese numbers.

"And what is the number of your apartment?" the woman asked me next.

"Eight C," I stated clearly. Glad I had finally memorized this. "Ba C."

The two officers paused and glanced at each other. The elevator bell rang, and its doors opened to swallow us whole. I felt as if I were in one of those human-interest stories I'd read in the state-run *Daily*—naïve foreigner who doesn't keep her visas straight ends up in hot water. I moved to step into the elevator and waited for the officers to follow. Who knew how this would play out upstairs, but it would be complicated. And involve my trying to explain in limited Chinese why I didn't have my registration papers or my passport or a copy of our resident permit or the original of Tony's work permit. In every scenario I was at fault.

Then for some reason, the male officer announced, "It's okay" to his partner and nodded at her. "Ba C," he said loudly for emphasis. *Ba C.* And maybe it was because they trusted my face, but probably not. More likely it was because living in an apartment numbered eight, China's luckiest number, means good luck will find you. This is how it happens every day inside China's quixotic system of rules. Maybe you're lucky. Maybe you're not. And you must learn to live within this arbitrary system and temper your *xiwang*—your urge to wish it was any different. Because in this story the officers both turned on their heels and walked out of Tower Five and left me standing inside the elevator alone while the automatic doors closed.

I'd like to say a few things now about Chinese permits. Because in China there are many of them: temporary resident permits and temporary work permits, long-term visas and short-term visas, visitor's permits and dog permits. Car permits and building permits. Even fireworks permits, though who bothers to get those is unclear. Here in China you need your long-term visa to get the temporary resident permit, and you need the lease agreement on your apartment in triplicate for the long-term visa. For the lease agreement you need copies of your passports, and then you take the stamped agreement to the nearest police station (after you find someone to direct you there, which may take days; the police station has moved), along with four wallet-sized photos. These photos must not be printed on white photo stock. They must be on blue stock. Don't think of going to the station if you've printed on white stock. The blue will get you that temporary resident permit you need. Because if you have that, you might be able to apply at the customs office for that stuff you packed up in boxes before you left the States. And by the time that shipment arrives in Beijing, you will have forgotten what you packed and why that stuff ever seemed important to you in the first place.

# II

# Hall of
# Mental
# Cultivation

交泰殿

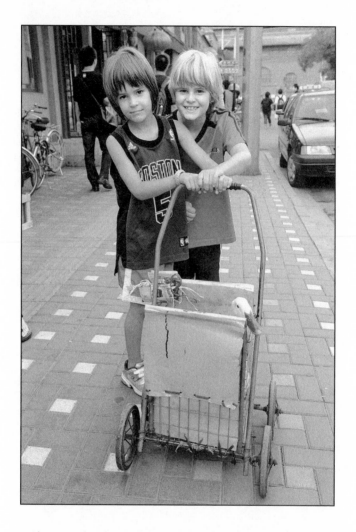

Thorne and Aidan in downtown Beijing in temporary custody of a duck who had come from the market in Houhai

# Houhai Lake

January 4, 2008. Aidan is five years old today. And how could that be? Almost five months have passed since we got to China. Tony and I take the boys to Houhai Lake to go skating. Lao Wu drives the van, and on the way Aidan says, "God is dead." Then he asks if he can have a lollipop. I remain silent on both fronts.

He repeats, "Did you know God was dead, Mom?"

"No, I didn't," I say in my most sunny voice. I'm looking out the window for something I can distract Aidan with—a big truck or a horse pulling a cart of watermelons. I'm not up for a talk about God. I want to discuss what being five years old means, and how proud Aidan must be that he can read picture books. "Who told you the news?" I finally ask him.

"A guy in my class read it in a book. A guy in my class read that God is dead," he adds for clarity. We're almost at the lake. "He died," Aidan explains one more time and then wraps up the conversation by asking Lao Wu directly for a candy. Which leaves me in the front seat pondering the state of the universe. I look back at Tony quickly to see how he's handling this information, but he's closed his eyes.

It's my suspicion that the boys have become more fascinated with death since we moved to China. Maybe it's just their age, or maybe China has clarified things for them—the grinding poverty, the chaos. Because the white-haired men who play cards across the street from our apartment near the cement shops lie down on the sidewalk for naps after lunch, and each time Thorne sees them, he asks me if the men have gone to heaven.

Here in China, God seems to have been dead for many years, and then recently brought back to life by the Chinese government. But if God is really dead, it doesn't seem to be bothering either of my children that much. We pull over in a crowded lane near the lake and get our skates out of the back of the van. I say nothing more about God and his demise. The lake is in the middle of Old Beijing, circled by teahouses and brick temples and stone courtyards. I stand on the street and look at the brick lanes leading out from the lake and feel the history. I could walk down one of those lanes and get lost for hours.

To skate on the lake, we pay fifteen RMB each to a short man in a stall over by a cluster of skinny benches. We get Thorne and Aidan laced up first, and when Tony is ready the three of them head out on the ice. I teeter down the ramp to the lake trailing after them, but I've forgotten to remove the plastic skate guards on my blades and fall flat on the ice. I'm not the only one trying to stand up. It looks like many first-timers. Lots of teenage girls hold hands and squeal. Aidan and Thorne link arms and begin skating faster and faster around the lake.

A few sharp-looking speed skaters circle in black one-piece suits. There are also men and women well into their sixties, who skate slowly and purposefully with broad smiles. They look so pleased. How could we not all be? A chocolate cupcake sits in the van for each of the boys. Later we'll sing "Happy Birthday" in Chinese to Aidan on the benches by the side of the lake. Right now it's a sunny Saturday in Old Beijing at the start of 2008. This city is seductive and God may or may not be dead, depending on whom you talk to.

On Sunday night, Tony and I go to dinner at a new Chinese fusion place with two couples we don't know—one of the husbands is a friend of a friend whose name we'd been given before we moved here. Sebastian. We're trying out a French babysitter named Chloé for the first time tonight. She's fifteen and lives in Tower Four with her brother, Arthur, a playground friend of Thorne's. She has her own cell phone and carries her laptop in a leather saddlebag, and the boys got her to play soccer in the hall within minutes of her arrival.

It's pitch-black inside the restaurant. Electronica plays in the background, and the ceiling lights are so low that I can barely make out my own place setting: white bowl on top of white plate, white chopsticks that sit on a small white ceramic bird. Sebastian is a tall, gray-haired man in his sixties, head of the Asian office of an international law firm. His wife, Margaret, sits next to Tony. She has striking black hair cut to her chin and says, by way of opening, that she's a psychiatrist at one of the international hospitals here. A man named Ned sits next to Sebastian. I put him at maybe thirty-five. He's got a completely bald head and an easy, engaging way. He runs the China office of a large investment bank. His wife, Elizabeth, sits next to me. Her blond hair is in a ponytail. She says she's just pulled off a birthday party for ten three-year-olds.

Everyone at the table wants Obama to win the U.S. presidential election, which is an icebreaker. But it's hard to talk because we can't see one another. A troupe of Chinese waitresses stands at attention along the back wall in black silk Chinese jackets. They serve thin slices of tuna on pink beds of radish and one sautéed shrimp wrapped in arugula. It's the new gourmet that's taken the country by storm—portions fit for children that cost more than the waitresses' combined monthly wages.

There's a worriedness to the way the waitress with the long ponytail keeps pouring more Shiraz for everyone. There's no ease to this restaurant, either. The chairs are hard and black. The floor is a dark shade of gray cement. I lean over to ask Margaret about her patients, and when my napkin falls, one of the girls is there at my knees to catch it and refold it for me. It turns out Margaret was one of the first Westerners in Beijing to practice psychiatry.

"My patients," she says, "are a mix of Chinese and foreigners. They and I do fine. It's more complicated with the hospitals here."

I tell her she should write a book. She laughs and says, "Psychiatry is so new here." And that she wishes she had more hours in the day.

Then Sebastian bangs his hand lightly on the table and says, laughing, "When is the real food going to arrive?"

Tony asks for the menu again. It's up to him to talk to the waitresses in Chinese and figure out more dishes. "Do you have any noodles?" I hear him ask in Mandarin. "Perhaps in a broth?" But this is a restaurant that has forsaken Chinese cooking and replaced it with a nouveau mélange of French finger food. And that's fine. I just wish the place didn't take itself so seriously here at the end of an ancient hutong alley, where people shuffle out in their pajamas to go to the public toilets around the corner.

I rise to find the bathroom, and a waitress hands me a flashlight. "Here," she says in broken English. "You will need this." I feel like I'm starting my solo on Outward Bound. I take the flashlight and head behind the tables down a long, black hallway that dead-ends in a wall of mirrors. The tiny flashlight doesn't give off enough light. Maybe I've had too much wine, because I'm unsteady and can't see more than one foot in front of me. I push on two different doors that don't open, and now I'm lost and the dining room is so dark no one will see that I'm missing.

I start to sweat, and then a door finally opens and I'm standing in a large, open room with a marble sink and toilet and hundreds of lit votives. The walls in the bathroom are covered from floor to ceiling in black bear fur. At first I can't believe it. I walk toward the wall with my arm outstretched. Then I turn around in a circle, counting how many bears must have been killed.

I sit to pee, but I feel like bears are watching me. It turns out I've had a lot of wine after all. I tell the bears that the New Beijing seems to have killed off the rest of their brethren. I go on to tell the bears how sorry I am. Then I stand and wash my hands and tell the bears I'm leaving. I make it back to the table, where Sebastian and Ned are laughing at a small collection of wasabi peas they've been handed on a Chinese saucer. More pretend food in this parallel universe. I hand the waitress my flashlight and she unfolds my napkin again and places it in my lap with a flourish.

Margaret asks Elizabeth what she's doing in Beijing and Elizabeth explains that she's writing a novel about the betrayal of her best friend by her husband when they were all expats together in London last year. My eyes widen. Someone else in the city who's trying to write a novel. "Tell me more," I say.

Elizabeth laughs. She's got a grin on her face. "Oh, I could. I could. But that's what I'm trying to do in the book. Let's just say there's a baby. And my friend isn't the mother." When I look closely at Elizabeth in the darkness, I can see that her eyes are a beautiful, icy blue. I don't know her well enough yet, or I would tell her what is going on back in that bathroom. Something about Old China meeting New. Something about bears and nature. It's definitely about darkness. About the darkness in this place.

# Human Migration

There's a snowstorm in central China this week and millions of migrant workers get stuck in train stations south of Beijing. The storm couldn't have come at a worse time. Tens of millions of Chinese are trying to get home for Chinese New Year. It's one of the greatest human migrations in the world, and whenever hundreds of thousands of angry citizens gather in public it's of concern to the Chinese government. More snow is predicted. The temporary shelters are full, and men have been sleeping out in the cold next to the tracks.

The way CNN International reports on the problem makes me think civil war is imminent. Their stories focus on tension at the train stations and the lack of food and water. My parents call on the phone from Mexico, where they've settled for a month. They get the same high-drama news, and they're certain that Beijing must be caught in the blizzards and that angry migrants are about to start a coup in Tiananmen.

Meanwhile, the sun shines down over Beijing, and we sit glued to our televisions to see what's going to happen down south. The migrant workers go home once a year to see their families. They don't seem to be budging until the trains come. But the trains can't come because the electricity grid is down.

Has anyone told the workers that? Or that China has not had this much snow in fifty years?

Rose comes for our Chinese lesson. She's put her hair up in a bun and wears an orange Donald Duck sweatshirt. What is it about Chinese fashion and American cartoons? Today I learn how to ask someone how their work is in Chinese: "Ni gong zuo hao ma?" The answer can be as simple as "Hao." *Good.* But there are other things you can say to answer, and here's where it gets confusing. You could say *hen hao* or *haixing* or *zenmeyang* or *bucuo* just for starters, and none of these words seems to have anything in common with the other.

In Mandarin the idea is often to turn the question around immediately: "Ni ne?" *And you?* Which is not so different from what we would do in English, so I'm happy to land for a moment on this parallel linguistics bar.

Then something exciting happens. Rose teaches me the Chinese verb *xiwang*. It means "to wish" or "to hope for," and this is the kind of verb that opens the language door wider for me. Because I've got all kinds of wishes since I moved to China. Different hopes for our life here. On smoggy days I wish it was sunny, and on sunny days I hope the smog stays away. I'd been beginning to wonder if the Chinese might have a lack of xiwang—an absence of hoping or wishing—because most of the sentences I'd learned were declaratives: "It *is* sunny" or "It *is* smoggy." I'd been beginning to think hoping and wishing was a Western construct. But now we've gotten to xiwang, and the country makes more sense. Because how could any nation live without hope?

The hour winds down, and Rose takes a sip of the warm water I've brought her. She says the Chinese never drink cold things and never use ice. The time at the end of our lesson has become my favorite part of the day in Beijing. It's when Rose describes pieces of her own life and switches, thankfully, into

English. She says that for the last two weeks she's been trying to buy a train ticket to go home for Chinese New Year. But they're sold out. "These men," she explains, "these bad men at the stations will sell me a ticket for ten times the real cost, but I don't have that kind of money."

"Wow." I stare at her. Communist scalpers. "I had no idea it was that hard to go home."

"It happens every year." She smiles. "You can only get home on the trains if you know someone. Or if you're willing to bribe." I'm thinking about my new verb *xiwang*, and wishing things with the ticketing might be changed. But Rose is a twenty-three-year-old in New China, with a cell phone and a bedroom in a group apartment in the capital. She has a college degree, speaks excellent English, and has prospered by problem solving within the system. "I have secured a ticket home from a friend of a friend of a friend," she explains. "He works on one of the trains leaving Beijing tomorrow. It's not really a ticket. It's a secret space on the train."

"But how will you get on?" I ask. "Won't the conductor see you?"

"The boy who works the train will smuggle me into the compartment early in the morning—when it's dark, before the others have begun to gather. I will bring American cigarettes to pay him off. All he wants is Marlboros."

"It sounds dangerous. And there's so much snow now. I don't think you'll get far. What will happen if the authorities find you?"

"They'll kick me off the train," she says. "But my parents are waiting for me. I am their only child. I see them once a year. I have to get back by the sixth."

This year on the sixth day of the month Chinese families will gather for dumplings and stay up until midnight to see in the new year. The night marks the end of the twelve-month lunar cycle and the beginning of the next. "The factories close," Rose explains, and takes another drink of water. "The shops shut down and everyone spends the day setting off fireworks."

"Why fireworks?"

"The Chinese love fireworks." She stands up from the couch. She has to go to her next lesson now. "Fireworks scare evil spirits away."

Later that night, I watch Prime Minister Wen on TV. He stands at a crowded train station to apologize to hundreds of thousands of workers camped out along the tracks. He says he's sorry for the weather—as if he's somehow responsible for the precipitation, and maybe he is. Or should be. Because I've begun to think that in this totalitarian by proxy government, the leaders can control the snow. One migrant worker interviewed blows his cool while people jostle him. "This government is terrible!" he yells. "The members of the party can go home for the holiday. But not the people. This government should be banned!" I wonder how long it took the secret police to find that man in the crowd.

Rose left on the train today, and I worry for her. It's snowed more in the south since I saw her, and crowds are trampling people at the train stations. Footage shows hundreds of thousands rushing at metal barricades at the train station in Guangzhou. It seems like maybe CNN was right—there really will be riots. The news reports that twenty-five people have died in a bus crash on a snowy highway.

Then the snow stops. Five days pass. The headline in the *China Daily* today reads, "Human strength prevails in the face of storms." Extra trains are brought in to take the workers home. Civil war gets averted. The *Daily* article profiles one older army official and the days of shoveling he did to rid a stretch of highway of freezing ice. The *Daily* is big on personal triumph stories. They also go in for accounts of sacrifice (death, maiming, disfigurement, or emotional toll) for the greater good of society. I keep wondering if Rose made it.

I finally call her on her cell phone and she answers right away. "It took me fifty hours on the train. I snuck inside the staff sleeping room and the boy gave me an engineer's uniform to wear."

"A uniform?" I ask. I can't believe what lengths she went to.

"Then I was told to lie still in the empty bed and pretend to sleep. I couldn't speak to anyone, and if someone asked me for a ticket, I was not supposed to open my eyes."

"I'm so glad you made it."

"I kept waiting for the train conductor to find me and kick me out into the snow. My parents were worried. But I'm here now. Eating like a pig and sleeping late. Tomorrow we go visit our cousins and eat at each house. It is the custom. We start with the oldest people and work our way down."

I ask if she thinks the government handled the storms well. "At first I thought no," she says into the phone. "I did a lot of reading on the Internet, and there everyone is angry at the government. But then I began talking to friends, and they persuaded me that the government couldn't control the weather."

I tell her I think the government could have warned the workers about the biggest snowstorm in fifty years. "They have computers that track storms, you know," I say. "They have Doppler radar."

"In the end the government did a good job of keeping the peace at the train stations," Rose says. "That is their job. To keep peace. You don't want people getting angry." I decide to drop it. Because maybe she's right. In any case, she's found a way to skip over the blame and to focus instead on the prime minister's last-minute solutions. Somewhere in this conversation there's a lesson for me in Chinese politics.

# Stuffed Like Mao

Now it's Chinese New Year week. Which means fifteen million Beijingren set off fireworks in the streets, and the city has become a pyrotechnic zone hard to exaggerate the scope of: hundreds of thousands of bottle rockets and air bombs and a thing I learned this morning is called a Chinese volcano. Makeshift fireworks shops have set up all over the city, and one of these metal sheds sits below our living room window. There are men you can hire down there to set your fireworks off for you if you're scared, or think explosives are beneath you. But you've got to buy the things and watch them get lit, even if you just stand by your car near the side of the road, because the only way you'll rid the next year of evil spirits is to witness each explosion.

Aidan woke at midnight last night crying, and we stood at his window watching the sky explode into multicolored rainbows until I convinced him to go back to bed. I'm not sure how anyone in this city sleeps. By the time Saturday comes around, we're tired of Chinese New Year. After breakfast we decide that for some reason today is the day to go see the Forbidden City.

We head out to the van and Thorne says "Zaoshang hao," to Lao Wu. *Good morning.* Inside the van Aidan leans against my shoulder, and Thorne lies down in the way back. Tony sits in the passenger seat. We set off, and I take the opportunity to read out loud from the guidebook: "Inside the Forbidden City the emperor was served over one hundred dishes at a time, but was only allowed two bites of each in case of poisoning." I don't think anyone in the van is listening. Or that anyone cares that we're going to see the most famous buildings in all of China—an ancient city within this ancient city, where the emperors lived with staffs of eunuchs. And where one poor concubine was drowned in a well.

Thorne climbs over the backseat and the boys begin arguing over who won the latest thumb-wrestling war. Then we hit a traffic jam on the stretch of Chang'an Jie Avenue near the south gate of the Forbidden City, but Lao Wu doesn't want to drop us off here. The real entrance, he tells Tony, is around the corner, past a giant, framed portrait of Mao that hangs on the wall. In the painting Mao's hair is combed to the side, and his skin looks polished. His eyes are unreadable.

Tiananmen Square sits across the next intersection of eight packed lanes of traffic. The square itself is an open arena, and Tony asks Lao Wu to loop us around so we can see the government buildings up close. They look like they've been imported from Moscow, circa 1972: cold and forbidding. Tony points to the right. "There's Mao's tomb."

"Where?" Thorne sits up quickly in his seat. "What is a tomb?"

Tony points again. "Mao's body sits in that building, right behind the square. Mao was the leader of China for a very long time."

"Is it really his body?" Aidan asks.

"It's his body," Tony says. "But it's not alive anymore. It's been preserved with chemicals."

"Kind of like a dead animal," I add. I can't think of any other way to explain it.

"Human taxidermy." Tony looks at me and smiles.

"Stuffed," Thorne says. "Mao's been stuffed. Just like the black bears downstairs at L.L. Bean."

"Well, kind of like that, but not exactly." Tony laughs. "Thousands of Chinese people line up to see Mao every day. I waited in that line." Tony looks over to the tomb again.

"You saw him?" Thorne can't believe it. "You saw Mao?"

The van is just to the west side of the tomb. "I didn't get to stay very long. There are guards who keep you moving. You never stand still. And you can't take photos."

"Do the guards have guns?" Aidan asks.

"They don't ever use them. I had to wait five hours. When I got close enough, I bought a bouquet of plastic flowers from a man near the tomb. After I saw Mao's face, a guard came and took the flowers from me and walked them back to the man so he could sell them again."

Tiananmen is the kind of space that plays tricks. It appears open and transparent, but if you look closer, you'll see the police vans: three unmarked white Buicks. What gives them away are the antennae on the roofs. These vans are ready to whisk you away should you be struck by the bad idea to start calling for regime change. Or if you get down on your knees in the square to pray. From what I've heard, the police are on you in seconds. They lift you off the ground and stash you in the van before other tourists register what's happened.

I ask Tony to ask Lao Wu if he has seen Mao's body. "Dui, dui," Lao Wu answers. He tells Tony he saw Mao in 1976, just after he died. Everybody had to go, he says. All the work units in Beijing took the day off to wait in line. It's impossible for me to guess what Lao Wu thinks of Mao. He goes silent again behind his poker face: his deep-set eyes give nothing away.

Then he's talking again. He tells Tony that everyone heard the gunshots. Everyone knew what was going on in Tiananmen in June of 1989. Tony nods and translates. Lao Wu says an army tank chased him home on the highway, with its machine gun pointed down at his window. He'd been out in the countryside on a delivery job, and he'd come back to the city unaware that the army had taken over the square.

Then just as quickly as he began talking, Lao Wu is quiet again. There's nothing more for him to say. He slows the van and lets us off with a smile. Two strangers on the sidewalk point at the boys and ask in English, "Two boys? You got two? Good work." We cross a moat and arrive at a small square in front of the ticket booth. It's crowded with hundreds of tour groups and guides who hold up different-colored flags and scream in Mandarin into handheld megaphones.

It's warm for late January in Beijing, maybe forty-five degrees Fahrenheit. We enter through two tall red gates and walk into the enormous courtyard. It takes a few moments for my eyes to adjust to the scale of the buildings and the mob of tourists. The courtyard is wide and long and much bigger than I imagined, with a red, lacquered hallway on either side that seems to run the length of the compound. In the middle of the yard is the Hall of Supreme Harmony, resplendent in shiny red paint. We cannot go inside, but we stand at the dirty windows and peek at an old kang and several high-backed wooden chairs in a big, dark room.

"I'm thirsty," Thorne says and sits on the side of the stairs. Then we walk on. The next courtyard leads to the Hall of Central Harmony.

"I'm tired," Aidan says next. I look at a map posted on the wall and it doesn't take long for me to realize how many more courtyards and pagodas and palaces await us: the Hall of Preserving Harmony, the Hall of Heavenly Peace—each amazing architectural feat following the next. And who really lived here? What was it like to take a nap in the Hall of Literary Glory? Or a meal in the Palace of Union and Peace?

Tony says we have to pick up the pace. "I'll race you to the next set of stairs," he calls out to Thorne, and then they're off, with Aidan sprinting to catch up. We make it through half the city like this—racing from landing to landing, going back in Chinese time. Then we break for Cokes at the café installed for tourists like us who are wondering if their kids will make it to the other side. There's a gift shop next door that sells fake vintage Mao alarm clocks and ceramic sculptures of Mao saluting. There are Mao T-shirts and Mao postcards. Mao stuffed dolls. Mao is a cottage industry here—it's one great big uneasy shopping trip. Didn't the Cultural Revolution end just thirty-four years ago?

Some of the staircases have stone ramps worn smooth over hundreds of years, and the new game that gets us through the second half of the Forbidden City is climbing to the top of each ramp and sliding down on your sneakers. Sneakers or bums, Aidan decides after he falls and makes it the rest of the way down on his bottom. We finally make it out and walk away from the crowds until we find a fast-food place around the corner.

It's China's version of McDonald's called Yummy's: a packed dining hall with rows of plastic tables and an all-you-can-eat Chinese buffet. Chicken tendons. Chicken feet. Chicken heads. The boys keep getting up for more chicken fried rice and fried chicken spring rolls. I drink some apple juice from a soda dispenser. We're the only foreigners here. I didn't know there were so many fat people in China, all crammed into their seats while a hostess with a headset on tells the long line of people that tables will be available soon. Tony picks at a few fried chicken drumsticks, and when the boys are finished I ask them to never talk me into coming to Yummy's again.

After lunch Lao Wu drives up to the curb in front of Yummy's and slows just enough in the moving traffic so we can all jump into the van. I'm hoping to go to this homemade-yogurt shop I've read about that's deep in the hutong. On the way Thorne wants to hear a story about my grandfather. "Why him?" I ask with my eyes closed.

Thorne loves to hear family stories. "Please tell me about Nona's father again."

My grandfather was a stern dad who morphed into a soft grandfather willing to build a series of rabbit hutches out of chicken wire in our backyard. He always went to church and belted out hymns, but he rarely seemed satisfied with the preacher. His last twenty years he typed a weekly letter, mimeographed so his four kids and eleven grandchildren could read his views on the state of American politics (appalled) and his hopes for his pruned bonsai (high). Named Albert Lewis Edgerton Crouter at birth, he went by many aliases: Sandy and Alec and Big Al and Opa. He was Gimpy to me. I'd call him from California and he'd yell into the receiver, "Hold the phone! Hold the phone. You're actually living in that godforsaken state? Judas Priest, girl. Why did you move so far from home?" But I think he was happy to know I was the traveling kind.

I sit up in the van and tell Thorne, "Every night when he visited, Gimpy would tell me a story about a horse named Mr. Snodgrass and two mice who lived under a general store with their parents."

"And he's dead now?"

I had a feeling this question was coming. I say yes and close my eyes again and hope that's the end of it. I want to rest. Why didn't any of the guidebooks mention that the Forbidden City is not kid-friendly?

"Did Gimpy get put in a grave or thrown in the water?"

Thorne asks. I open my eyes and he's staring at my face. It must be Mao's tomb that's sparked them.

Then Aidan leans over and says, "Yeah," as if he's been part of the conversation all along. "If Gimpy was put in a grave, then we can visit him." This is Aidan's way—to be sanguine about the big stuff. It's the small stuff that sometimes snags him.

"He has a gravestone in Vermont," I say. That much I know is true. When my grandfather retired, he and the Madame lived full-time in a wooden house on Lake Champlain, where they canned beets and fished for trout with worms. Vermont was their holy land.

"Mommy," Aidan says now and takes my hair in his hand. "When it's time, you can choose a gravestone, and then we can come and visit. We'll just move the stone over and look down at you."

"Not exactly," I say slowly. We're in deep here. "You can't really move the stone."

This is when Thorne announces, "I don't want to be buried. I want to be stuffed. I want to be stuffed just like Mao."

"Yes," Aidan says. "Stuffed like Mao."

Before I decide whether to laugh out loud, Lao Wu pulls the van over in the alleyway near the yogurt shop. There are four flavors to choose from today: vanilla, wheat germ, almond, and pistachio. Tony orders one of each and we carry the bowls to the one open table. It's a light, creamy yogurt, and we all want more, so Tony rises for another round. The line now reaches out the door. After he's eaten his second bowl, Aidan has to pee, so he and Tony walk outside to find a public squatter toilet.

Thorne and I finish our second yogurts and then he asks for one more. "You like it that much?" I say, and I hand him the coins and watch him stand in line. Six months ago he would have balked at the idea of waiting with strangers in a

Beijing yogurt shop. Now he gets to the counter and I hear him ask in Chinese which one is coffee-flavored. When he and I step out into the midday haze, bottle rockets are zinging in the alleyway behind us.

Aidan rounds the corner. "Mom, Mom. You've got to come! You won't believe this." Thorne and I follow him around the yogurt shop, where Tony kneels on the ground with three Chinese men, trying to light a fistful of sparklers. They're the long kind I've never let the boys handle before. The dangerous sparklers. But then they're lit, and the men hand one to each of us, and the men's wives come out of the house now with a whole other bag of fireworks and everyone is laughing and waving sparklers in the air.

I'd heard that for years the government banned fireworks in Beijing because of the danger, but the outcry from the people was too great. I watch one of the men bend to light another bottle rocket with a lit cigarette dangling from his lips. Each time there's an explosion the sound echoes off the stone houses and careens back. I put my hands over my ears. One of the men gives Thorne the lighter and motions for him to set off the next round. I'm over by the doorway—trapped in a parenting moment deep in the cultural vortex. I could yell out, "No!" and insert myself, explaining that my kids don't play with fire. I could say that fire is dangerous. Or I could just be quiet and let this unfold.

It's a learned skill for me—this notion of stepping back. Of dropping into that Daoist river. But it's also something China demands. I have a small camera in my bag, and I take it out. I'm able to capture Thorne as he bends down close to the bottle rocket with the cigarette lighter. Tony is beside him. Aidan is to Tony's left, and the trio of other men is next to Aidan. I take more pictures. It helps me to stay busy. Even the wives lean in close now—trying to explain to Thorne how to light the thing. Through the camera lens Thorne looks scared. I'm not sure my son wants to be doing this. But I do not say one word. And then it's done and the rocket hisses and burns and zings in the sky above us. I glance up quickly and then back over to Thorne. I could swear he's standing a little taller—and that he's wearing one of those small, private smiles, imperceptible perhaps to everyone but his mother.

# The Three T's and the One F

Today the Internet says two hundred people are dead in Lhasa and Tibetan monks have taken to the streets. We can't get any YouTube footage of the riots in Beijing. Each time I click on a photo of the fighting in Lhasa, my computer screen goes blank. It's an unsettling feeling—as if some government censor has gotten inside the apartment and is standing in my bedroom, leaning over my shoulder. What's really happened is that by typing in the word *Tibet,* I've tripped an alarm on an Internet filter at the government's mother ship.

The Chinese have kicked foreign journalists out of Tibet and are bringing tanks into Lhasa today. These edicts come down just a mile or so from our apartment, in the government compound that circles Tiananmen, but Tony's and my lives go eerily unchanged. It's an odd thing to be so close to the mechanisms of war, but to learn about them only in stolen Internet moments.

We meet Sebastian and Margaret for dinner again—this time at a Yunnan place called South Seas. Their friends Gwynne and Alex join us. Chloé has come to babysit for the second time, and the boys have planned a badminton tournament with her in Aidan's room. Gwynne is a petite woman with shocking blue eyes and a great, throaty laugh.

She says she's here to research Internet use. When she puts out her hand to greet me she asks, "Has anybody been able to get on the BBC Web site since the protests started in Tibet?" Her husband, Alex, is a journalist for an American magazine.

I sit next to Gwynne at the square wooden table, and during dinner she tells me she's learned there are four things you can't talk about in China. "They're called 'the Three T's and the One F,'" she says. "Tibet, Taiwan, Tiananmen, and Falun Gong. Bringing up any of these topics"—she smiles and takes a sip of beer—"will not win you any friends in the Chinese government."

I keep looking over my shoulder, wondering if any of the waitresses here are spies, but no one seems to be paying us any attention. "Do you ever worry about your husband in China?" I ask Gwynne after we've polished off a small plate of garlic and mushrooms.

"I worry about Alex, but never about the things I should be worried about. And right now he can't get a flight to Lhasa. No one can."

"I read today that the protests have spread over Yunnan," Sebastian says. "And that monasteries are organized all across China."

"Good luck and Godspeed," Margaret says then. "I feel like this is the Tibetans' last stand before the Olympics. Their last chance for world attention."

Gwynne nods. "Did you know that when the government here isn't busy shutting down Web sites about Tibet, it's trying to control the speed of our Internet search engines? Take this week, for example; they've ratcheted things down so that even if you get on a sanctioned Web site, you won't want to stay because it's so slow."

"So that's why Yahoo has been creeping along," Tony says.

"And they don't do it to punish anyone, just to make sure everyone knows they're there, watching," Gwynne adds.

When Tony and I get back to the apartment after dinner, the restaurant outside our bedroom still has the lights on. It's a long, low family place with big picture windows. If we look closely, we can see the noodles people eat for dinner. We go into the living room and Tony turns on CNN. We get five seconds of Lhasa riot footage before the screen goes dead again. We switch to the BBC. It's blacked out too. "I can't believe they do this!" Tony yells. "As if we won't get our news somewhere else."

But I'm thinking about what Gwynne said—that this kind of censorship slows down information access to the point where we give up trying. It makes things just difficult enough tonight so we go to bed early. Tony and I lie under the sheets. There is the sound of a small electric drill in the ceiling above us. We're never sure if our apartment is bugged. Tony and I aren't important enough for that. Still, earlier today the property management office called and said maintenance men would be over again to "fix some problems with the air-conditioning." These "problems" are confusing to us—the AC has worked fine since the first week. Tony and I hold hands and fall asleep listening to the sounds of hammering in the air duct.

On Monday morning Rose and I take our class to the giant IKEA home goods store just off the Fourth Ring Road North. I need to find a mattress pad. The hard Chinese bed we sleep in has begun to bruise my back. Rose would like to buy a coffeepot. She's never been to IKEA before. She meets me at the front door of Tower Five with a big smile. She says her boyfriend wants to know what she's buying before she pays for it.

We get in the van with Lao Wu and I ask her, "Do you think the Chinese army is being too forceful in Tibet?" I've been waiting to pose this question all weekend.

"Susan, the Chinese army is just doing its job." I look out the window and wonder how much Rose really knows. Then she says, "Tibet has always been part of China." She views the protests in terms of how much danger they pose to the Chinese people. "The army has to keep the peace in Tibet, Susan. Tibetans are killing Han." Then she says she's more worried about the Olympics. "I saw a fortune-teller last week who told me that during the games there will be blood in the Beijing streets."

Lao Wu lets us off inside the parking garage, and we take the escalator to the third floor, which is stocked with aisles of sleek Swedish furniture: maple platform beds and stainless-steel desks. I'm surprised again at how many people are in China—how many men and women wheel shopping carts in and out of the Marimekko bedroom displays. It's the same IKEA stuff, but tweaked for the China market: smaller beds, and chopsticks in the kitchenware aisle.

Rose holds up a red French coffee press and calls out, "What is this?"

I leave my cart and circle back to her. "It's for coffee," I explain and take it from her. "You put the coffee in and then you press down like this."

"My boyfriend enjoys coffee now." Rose smiles. "More Chinese like coffee. But I do not think he would like this item."

There are maybe fifty different kitchen contraptions displayed on a grid of white shelves along the wall. Next Rose picks up a metal whisk. "And this?"

"For cooking," I say. "For beating eggs." Rose looks confused. "It's called a whisk," I say. "To stir things quickly."

She gazes at the gadgetry. "There is so much here," she says. "So much I don't see the use of."

She puts the whisk in her shopping cart and holds up a bright green garlic press. "Garlic press," I say. "You don't need it."

Next is an orange plastic spatula. "Do you like pancakes?" I ask her. She stares at me for a second too long, and I realize she doesn't know this word *pancakes*. Sometimes I forget that Rose has never left China. Or maybe never seen pancakes. I can't decide what she makes of this place and the well-heeled Chinese milling in the designer lighting aisle.

"Who are you buying this stuff for?" I ask her. "Yourself or your boyfriend?"

She smiles. "I'm not sure yet." When we get to the tall pyramid of Chinese woks, Rose is unimpressed. "Those woks are cheaply made," she says. "The iron is too thin."

"Shall we go to bedding?" I say quickly. Then I catch myself. "Shall we go find where they keep the mattress pads?" She nods and we wheel our carts away from the buzz of so many people shopping. The hallway is wide and relatively empty. I know Rose isn't interested in talking any more about Tibet. She wants to find the shower curtains. And I wonder if most people in this store are as apolitical as Rose seems.

*We Chinese believe in ourselves. We believe in our things.* Rose's boyfriend calls her on her cell for the second time since we've gotten to IKEA. She talks to him for two minutes, then hangs up. "He is jealous that we are here," she says. "He does not want me seeing these things for the first time without him."

# I Love You.
# End of Discussion.

On Sunday I take a yoga class. It's part of my self-enhancement plan: more women friends. More stretching my calves and quieting my mind. It's me and a teacher named Mimi. Her dark hair hangs down to the waist of her wide-legged pink pants. We sit on the floor of a white room in her apartment. It took me forty minutes to walk here, and I already feel better for having come. Mimi thinks we should start slowly. I haven't done the postures for years and my back feels stiff and unyielding.

She has me stand in front of the wall and press against it with both arms. I hold the pose while she instructs me on how I might begin to breathe differently—slower, filling up my rib cage with air. Then she asks me to bend toward the floor. She has a relaxing voice and an easy, comfortable way. She reminds me how to lower myself gently into a pose called Cobra and then says I'm stronger than I think I am. She tells me she was born in the States but her parents are Chinese. Now almost her whole family is living in China again.

By the end of our hour I can tell that Mimi is one of those gifted teachers you're lucky to meet in any lifetime. I stand to leave and my body feels looser. My mind has less chatter. I can also touch my toes again. I sign up for a series of Wednesdays and walk home feeling lighter.

*I Love You. End of Discussion.*

The streets around Mimi's house are a rare grid of roads still drawn to pedestrian scale: food kiosks and fruit carts line the sidewalks. The city feels alive. I can smell the garlic and hear the bike vendor calling out about his meat for sale.

At home I make a dinner date with a woman named Molly. She and her husband, Dan, and their two-year-old, Ann, moved here from California six months before we landed. They live one apartment complex down from us, in Palm Springs. Dan is in charge of an online photo Web site. He lived in Hong Kong for five years and speaks mean Chinese. Molly is a fearless traveler and businesswoman—busy now taking care of Ann. She and I met for coffee last week, at which point she was patient enough to draw me a detailed map of our neighborhood, highlighted with the places I might be able to buy an iron.

On Friday our families walk to the Lotus Blossom—a Buddhist restaurant that sits at the end of a garbage-filled alley twenty minutes from our apartment. Buddha statues appear along the alley to mark the way. Some of us are hungry when we make it to the Lotus Blossom. Some of us under the age of seven are cranky. There's another Buddha statue standing by the restaurant door, this one life-sized. Inside, the waiters are bald monks who wear gray cotton tunics and pantaloons and hover around our table handing out warm washcloths on bamboo trays.

Our place mats are gigantic palm fronds. We're hoping to order quickly—maybe noodles and dumplings. Molly says, "We need to get these kids fed." I nod to her as a waiter hands me the menu. It's a bound book the size of Aidan. I reach out and hold it with two hands and try not to giggle.

I rest the menu partly in my lap and open it to the first

page. Every dish has been given a "Buddhist poem name" to help inspire our order. There are no simple noodle dishes. No dumplings. This is going to be a more complicated meal than we planned. We try to study the menu—the kids are hungry and fidgeting and the book is so big. I finally tell Tony, "I'm ordering a dish called 'I love you. End of discussion.'" And then I do giggle. The names are too good.

Dan says, "I'm getting 'Contemplating the Inner Self Spinach.'" His laugh is this great, unexpected, raucous thing.

Then Molly announces, "For me 'Chinese Kale: A Little More Love, a Little Less Misfortune' and 'The Heart Has No Hang-Ups Palmelo Salad.'"

Tony and Dan together pick "No Birth No Death Tofu" and "In Praise of Going in Happiness Wild Yams." They also order Buddhist virility drinks made with smashed yams that are supposed to invigorate their sperm.

The food takes a long time to prepare. Aidan stands up on his chair and asks for more orange juice. At one point Ann is singing. I reach for Tony's virility drink. It tastes like sweet potatoes. Thorne keeps shredding his palm frond place mat. I'm able to distract him by taking him to the bathroom, where flute music is piped in on speakers and the sink is filled with stones.

When we get back to the table, Tony takes Aidan outside to stand on the porch the monks have built in the alley. "There are stars out there!" Aidan says when he returns. "Stars and candles!" The food arrives and somehow we've managed to order well: tofu and fake duck and fake chicken. We scoop glass noodles from one of the soup broths and sell them to the children. Everything is delicious. We eat quickly, and when the bill comes, we hand over wads of cash from our wallets, then walk back to the alleyway.

"Stars!" everyone says almost in unison. Aidan was right. The sky is clear and the night is dark.

"Mom!" Thorne yells. He is standing next to one of the Buddha statues, and he and the Buddha are the same height. "Mom! We are in outer space!" Then he begins laughing. "Right this very second the Earth is spinning in outer space!" Somehow standing in this dark alley in downtown Beijing on a Sunday night in February has unlocked a secret of the universe for my seven-year-old. Maybe China has allowed him to see the sky more clearly. I think all four of us have better vision here.

"Pretty cool, huh?" I squeeze Thorne's hand, and we begin to walk toward the end of the alley and the taxicabs. "Outer space. Pretty cool."


When we get home, Thorne lies down in his bed, and I pull the sheets up around his chin and rest next to him. This is when he asks me if I'm going to die soon. What he says exactly is, "Are you going to die in China?"

"No," I say, and press my face into his neck. "Not planning on it." I think the ties that bind us feel tighter here. Or maybe it's that we need to articulate them more in China. And what a nice surprise—that the world has slowed down enough for us to name our affections. But hard questions come more often from the boys in Beijing. They seem to lie at the surface.

"What if you die in a taxicab?" Thorne asks me next. "What if you die while I am at school?" I hug him and tell him I won't die for almost a hundred years. Almost forever. It's my standard answer. I've been told there are kids who don't explore the depths of their existential dread but my kids always have. I think China has given them a bigger frame for the story. A clarity of vision they didn't always have in the States.

"Almost to infinity is when I'll die," I whisper to Thorne.

I unwrap his arms from my neck and say I'll be right back with Daddy. Then Tony lies down with Thorne, and in minutes I hear them both laughing about the ace Red Sox closer Jonathan Papelbon, and what his earned run average was last September. Thorne talks to me about death and laughs about baseball stats with Tony? What is it with mother love? Why does it get so heavy?

Aidan is still awake. He keeps calling for me from the bottom bunk. "Which god do you believe in?" he asks when I get there. Couldn't we just go to sleep? Aidan's been asking me this question every day this week.

"Which one do you believe in?" I volley. I don't want to have to find another way to explain that I'm not sure what I believe. That I'm still figuring it out like he is. I explain that the Native Americans believed in animal gods and that Buddhists believe in the Buddha and that people called Christians believe one god did all the work.

Aidan announces, "I believe in the one god. And I believe in Jesus Christ, too. Jesus was a good man." I stare down at my child. "They nailed Jesus to the wall," he says then. "They nailed him and he died."

I had not planned on talking about Christ's sacrifice tonight. What I want to do is lie down in my bed and read. But I need to set the record straight. "Aidan," I say, and smile nervously. "Aidan, I believe Jesus was a nice man, too. That he was a very good man. But where, by the way, do you talk about Jesus?" I try to sound casual. "At school?"

I hope his answer will be no. Because we will have a problem if the secular international school in Beijing is dipping into religion. "Not at school. Just talking," Aidan says. "Just talking with friends. Which god do you believe in, Mommy?" He won't let it go. Then he makes an abrupt shift of course and says, "Mommy, who will be the next wife when you die?"

I've been working on trying to be patient in China. On trying not to be a helicopter mom. There's a small boy in bed with big, brown eyes and he's lying on his stomach with his bottom up in the air. He used to sleep like that when he was a baby. I'd come into the room to check on him in his crib, and his little tush would hang suspended above his legs. I put my hand out now and gently flatten his body on the sheet. I can't help that I find his question unfeeling.

I know he doesn't mean it, but is this really my son? Daydreaming about an imaginary new mother while I have spent afternoons worrying over the state of his psyche and whether or not his Spider-Man costume was clean? I'm thinking of a way to change the subject. And once we're done here, I'll have to dig out the Brazelton parenting book and see how long the fascination-with-death stage is supposed to last. Because Aidan has to know a second mommy requires something to happen to the first. Or maybe he hasn't thought it through that far? "I have some good ideas for the next mommy," Aidan says and closes his eyes.

# III

# Hall of Martial Valor

# 交泰殿

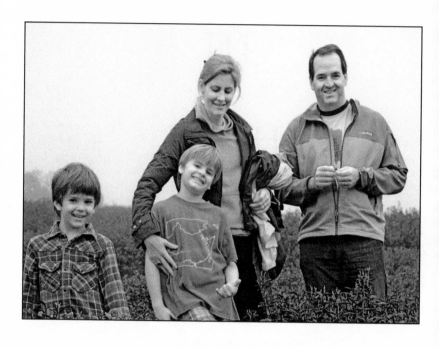

Tony, Susan, Thorne, and Aidan in the tea fields of Hangzhou, in Zhejiang Province

# Tell Me in Centimeters

By the time we're crowded into the ultrasound room together, spring has come to Beijing. It's April now, and the Chinese surgeon is here, and the Chinese radiologist, and Tony and me. Everyone is speaking loud Mandarin, which forces Tony to concentrate on what they're saying. I found the lumps myself the week before. It was a Sunday morning, and I was talking with the boys in bed about whether or not we'd go swimming. I leaned up against the pillows and made small circles with my index finger under my collarbone. I often do this. I wasn't checking for anything, just listening to the boys tell me how much they wanted to practice the backstroke and could we go now please?

The lumps felt like marbles. Two of them. I showed them to Tony after the boys left to get their swimsuits on. "Feel this," I said. "Does this seem weird to you?" And he said the perfect thing, which was that he was sure the lumps would go away on their own, but maybe I should make an appointment anyway.

A week later, the lumps still felt like marbles. That's what the Canadian internist told me when she felt my chest at the Beijing international hospital—that we were looking for marbles. Marbles or peas. I thought I'd hit the jackpot. But none of these people watching the ultrasound takes me seriously. The Chinese radiologist works quickly and takes the requisite pictures. "There's one," I say into the TV screen while everyone looks. "And there's the other." We all agree that there are lumps on the screen—that's no longer in dispute. But what's *inside* the lumps? One by one, the doctors in the room say the lumps are *nothing to worry about. Leave them alone and check again in three months.* I think it's a Chinese nervous thing—these patronizing smiles. Because I don't understand what it is we're smiling about.

The radiologist speaks English that's blunt and formal. I suspect he has a narrow bandwidth of English vocabulary in which to discuss breasts. And I don't blame him for that, but the effect is stern and dismissive. "These are tiny masses," he reminds me. "These are nothing." This country doesn't seem big on patient advocacy. This is the top-down model—doctor knows best.

I stare again at the little smudges on the screen that he's located with his probe. They are small; he's right. "But how do we know they're nothing?" I ask. I'm not really worried yet. I'm just aiming for due diligence. As a rule, I do not fret about my health. Up on the TV my entire left breast looks suspect—grainy and textured and alien. But everything appears foreign with ultrasound. My own babies' heads looked like exaggerated Martian skulls when I first saw them on the sixteen-week ultrasound.

"How do we know they're harmless?" I repeat. Because the lumps are small, but they're also in the middle of my breast, and what are they doing there? The radiologist doesn't answer. It's as if he hasn't heard me. Then I realize he may not have understood my question. I have a bad habit in China of speaking English too fast. "So we're not worried?" I say again, more slowly this time, and sit up on the examining table. "We're not doing anything about these right now?"

"These cysts are tiny," the radiologist repeats and hands me a tissue to mop up the goop he's spread on my chest with the probe. "The cysts are fluid. There's nothing that's worrying me about the cysts."

I reach for my shirt, and the surgeon, Dr. Lan, smiles knowingly at me again. "Tiny," he says, echoing the radiologist. "They are tiny cysts. Too small to take out." Then he does something I'll never forgive him for. He hands me a small wooden ruler. "Tell me how big you think your lumps are," he demands, and grins. "On the ruler. Tell me in centimeters."

I look at him and then over at Tony, and I'm confused. My eyes fill with tears. I haven't come to the ultrasound room to argue about how big the lumps in my breast are. I want to make a run for it. I want to leave this zooey hospital with its condescending smiles and rulers.

The problem is, Dr. Lan seems to be the only breast expert in town. The other problem is the ruler he gives me is in centimeters. I've never learned the goddamn metric system, so I can only think of my lumps in terms of inches. "I don't know," I say and stare at Tony while the tears fall. I have a funny feeling in my stomach—like something is not right. Something is not adding up in this examining room. If I keep my eyes locked on Tony, it makes it easier to speak. "I have no idea how big the lumps are in centimeters."

"Well," Dr. Lan says in his labored English, "the lumps on the ultrasound are much smaller than the way you described them at first." Then he adds, "I see these all the time on young women like you and they're nothing. Besides"—he pauses now and begins harping on the scar issue again, something he'd brought up in his examining room before he'd walked me over to radiology—"there will be a scar. And if you're like most Chinese women I know, you do not want a scar, do you?"

I look at him and wonder if he's been listening to me at all this afternoon. I do not care about scars. I'm not a single Chinese woman trying to find a mate. I've been married fifteen years and have two small boys. I do not give one flying fuck about scars. "You should wait," the surgeon repeats, and for some reason he keeps smiling. "Even if you are a worrier, you should wait. Are you a worrier? You should wait and check back with me in three months."

It is decided. We will wait.

How it goes after this is I call my doctor in the States. "Wait? How long 'wait'?" says Dr. Rainville. It's nine o'clock in the morning in Portland, Maine.

"Three months 'wait,'" I say loudly over the phone. The line from Beijing is scratchy.

"We never wait. I never advocate waiting." Dr. Rainville is a woman who doesn't mince words.

"No?" I ask. I am calling her from my bed, and now I put my head down on my pillow and close my eyes. I was afraid she might say this. Afraid my time with Dr. Lan in Beijing was not over yet.

"No waiting. Because you can't be sure, Susan. No waiting. You go in and you find out."

I call Dr. Lan back the next morning. "It's Susan," I say into the phone after a nurse tracks him down. "The American with breast lumps. I'm not waiting. I can't wait."

The thing is, in China, if you have money you can undergo surgery any day you want. There's no backlog at the international hospital, and so the very next morning I'm scheduled in the operating room at ten. Before Tony and I go, Aidan climbs into bed and lies between us and asks if we'll live in China forever. It's still dark out and the dump trucks are quiet in the hutong. Tony says no—there'll come a day when we move back to the States. Then Aidan says, "I like it here. It is different than Portland. There is bamboo in China." Which gets me wondering again how the mind of my five-year-old works. Mostly, I've decided, Aidan lives in a kind of free association: one thought leads to another until they can be strung together to form a series. How nice to live in that nonlinear space—a land of sights and smells and memories and no breast surgery.

What will transpire between now and then is I'll feed the boys Honey Nut Cheerios and poached eggs. Then I'll go over Thorne's spelling words with him (this week he has compounds like *chopstick* and *crossroad*). I'll fill each boy's backpack with a water bottle and a bag of Wheat Thins for the bus ride home. Then Tony will walk the boys down to the bus stop. I won't tell them I'm having surgery today. At the door, just before they go, I'll say, *Have a great time at school. You know how much I love you.*

If neither boy looks me in the eye, I'll say it again: *You know, right? You know how much I love you?* I can do this now that I'm having surgery. I can push the envelope on how much you talk openly about the love with elementary-school boys. And sometimes Thorne can be harder to get my hands on, but there he is, standing in the elevator, smiling at me while I kiss him one last time. Aidan drinks it up. He's always open to talking about the love and how much—just as long as it isn't *in public.*


At the hospital, the nurse walks me into an examining room to have an EKG before the surgery. They are big on EKGs in China. I've already had two here (which is two more than I'd had in my whole life before now). For some reason the Chinese feel EKGs are the benchmark for good health. You can't get a long-term visa here until you've passed your EKG. You might have some serious disease (like cancer, for instance, or hepatitis) and they'll let you into the country, but not if you have a weak EKG.

The nurse has trouble with the machine's wires, which are connected to small round suction cups meant to adhere to the skin on my chest, but they've lost most of their sucking power. When things seem to be in place, I lie back on the bed while Tony watches from a chair across the room. The machine spits out numbers on the ream of graph paper and then the nurse turns to me in alarm. She asks loudly, in a heavy Chinese accent, "Are you having heart attack? Do you feel unusual?" Her words are labored and rushed. Tony stands up and grabs the graph paper and looks over at me. Then he reaches for one of the little suction cups that's come loose on its wire.

"Do you feel unusual?" the nurse screams again, and I shake my head.

I want to tell her yes. *Yes, I do feel unusual.* I'm about to have breast surgery in China with an unwilling surgeon. I don't have family here, so while I'm in surgery, my children will be watched by our wonderful ayi, whose last name I am still a little unsure of. She lives in a small village out near the airport and I don't know the name of that either or what these lumps are doing inside my breast. The one thing I know on this Thursday morning is that I'm not having a heart attack. My heart feels fine.

After the EKG, the nurse walks me into a small changing room and hands me a hospital johnny made of green crepe paper. I put it on and come out into the waiting room and then I'm the naked woman standing in front of the bank of upholstered brown chairs, wearing a see-through gown. That's when I start laughing so hard I cry. Tony takes a picture of me wearing the thing, and then he laughs too, while I run back inside the changing room and wait for him to bring the nurse, who hands me something else to put on made of gray cotton.

"Who told you to put that on?" the new nurse asks in English with a straight face. Then she says, "Ha. Funny. That's funny. Take it off now."

When the surgery is over, we have to wait for the pathology in a post-op room where there's sledgehammering going on. I'm not alone in this room—a sweet-faced seven-year-old Chinese boy lies behind the curtain next to me. He keeps screaming in pain—long, sustained, high-pitched screaming. How has it come to be that my boys are at home, oblivious to my surgery, while there's a little boy Aidan's age next to me, going through his own hell? Tony sits on the bed, holding my hand, looking more and more worried. The pathology is taking too long. He has a bad feeling, I can tell.

What he explains to me later is that Dr. Lan burst out of the operating room after the surgery and told Tony the tissue looked funny. But Tony doesn't tell me this now. What he does is hold my hand and, every now and then, touch my face. The sledgehammering goes on, and Tony asks the nurse in Chinese what the problem is. It's as if men are pounding into the wall behind my head. It's impossible to sleep and hard to hear ourselves speak. The little boy's extended family comes and huddles around his bed. There are twelve of them—aunties and uncles and grandparents and parents. The boy's father finally takes the boy in his arms and rocks him to try to ease his crying.

147

We wait for the pathology some more, but I know now. I know because Tony is jittery, and he hardly ever acts this way, even though he hates hospitals. For years Tony went to the hospital in Hartford, Connecticut, with his sister, Polly, while she had her leukemia shots. He's told me the shots she got were scary big. It was the 1970s. Tony was eight, Polly was six. Most children didn't survive leukemia then. Tony would watch Polly get the shots and see how much pain she was in, and then he'd tell their mother he had a stomachache so he and Polly could stay home from school together. Tony missed a lot of school during those years.

Now he keeps standing up and pacing our little corner and then sitting down again and taking my hand. The boy next to me finally falls asleep. His family stays in the room, but they get quiet too. Then Dr. Lan must have come and fetched Tony because when I wake up, Tony is standing next to me, holding my hand and crying.

"It's bad," he says. "It's not good. It's bad." The first thing I think of is how silly we'd been to take those stupid pictures of me in the see-through green johnny. How carefree we were just three hours ago—and that we can never go back there. I believe that kind of laughter is lost to us now. The second thing I realize is that I've never seen Tony scared before. Never scared like now. He stands above the hospital bed and weeps, and it brings the whole thing home.

I'm awake and crying too and the sledgehammering below us is so loud. Is it coming from the walls? Where is it coming from? The little boy next to me begins to stir and that's when his father walks over to the nurse by the door and begins to rage in Chinese about the hammering and the inefficiency of the hospital and how could the place be so inept. He yells loudly until the little boy wakes up. Then Tony tells me that Dr. Lan won't let me go home. "He is deciding whether or not to go back in and do the mastectomy right now," Tony explains. "He's worried he's stirred up the cancer and that he needs to finish what he started."

"Mastectomy?" I whisper. How have we gone from harmless cysts to mastectomy? There's the sledgehammering in my head and the fact that Dr. Lan does not believe in doing needle biopsies and so I've had an unplanned lumpectomy. I realize later that Dr. Lan is not able to do needle biopsies. He does not know how. Then I have to remember that the Canadian internist told me I had a choice about whether or not to use this hospital. Dr. Lan was a good surgeon, she'd said, but they did not have a cancer program at the hospital. They did not engage in what we in the Western world call "patient care." I'd wanted to stay in Beijing for the surgery. I hadn't wanted to fly off to Hong Kong or Boston. What hit me was that Beijing had become my home. It had snuck up on me, but it was home now.

The little boy's father demands to see the hospital manager. Then Tony stands up again too, and together both men say they won't pay unless the nurse produces someone who can explain the noise. The nurse goes down into the bowels of the hospital and brings back some mid-level manager of something, who says in Chinese how sorry he is. Tony answers that you can't have surgery patients recovering in a construction zone. That they need to rest. They need sleep. It isn't fair.

And why? the boy's father asks. Why now? Why today? That is when the manager explains that the noise is because of the Olympics. "All the dignitaries and athletes will need extra rooms," he explains. "There will be injuries and dehydration. We are working around the clock—night and day—to finish the new construction," he says. "And we are behind."

Then Dr. Lan pops his head in through my curtain and

smiles. He says he's thinking it would be best to go back in and finish the surgery and proposes an on-the-spot mastectomy. He is trying, I decide, to make up for his nonchalance. "Get me out of here," I say to Tony in English. "You have to get me out of here."

# Inner Mongolia

Right now I'm in the bulkhead of Continental Airlines Flight 85 heading back to Beijing from Boston, where I've seen a small soccer team of doctors. The plane crosses the North Pole and heads out over the broad expanse of Russia. Dr. Lan got the initial cancer out—but in Boston I learned I have enough trouble to warrant the mastectomy. The next surgery is on the books in one month in Boston. One long month, and I haven't even landed in Beijing yet.

The man next to me on the plane owns a plastic bottle manufacturing plant. He looks like the actor Greg Kinnear's twin brother. He tells me his company makes every kind of plastic bottle you can imagine. "Spritzers," he says. "Pour tops, and bottles with caps, and water bottles. Any time you go into Walgreens," he says, "the plastic bottles in that store came from me." I smile at him. I've hit a new personal low, and I haven't found the bottom of it yet. We don't know how bad the cancer is. Won't know until after the next surgery. I'm sad and dazed by the travel and the litany of doctors. According to my Boston team, my cancer story is still a good one. *You caught it early* is the refrain I heard. It amazes me how cheery people can be about a cancer diagnosis.

Greg Kinnear seems nice. I don't have the heart to ask if

he's heard the recent news that plastic bottles are leaching into our food and disrupting our endocrine systems. Or that some researchers think plastics might be directly related to breast cancer. I watch *Atonement* on my own TV screen and cannot believe how sad a movie it is. I'm trying to be hopeful while I fly back across time zones and hemispheres. But if you admired the novel like I did, then you know the movie is going to be sad from the start.

I'm trying to be about good endings right now. But it's as if somewhere over Inner Mongolia, I hear the Boston surgeon's words for the first time: *mastectomy*. My kind brother, John, met me in Boston at the airport. Then he and my amazing friend Electa took notes in the white hospital rooms with the doctors. Every evening we'd gather in the cozy restaurant of my small hotel on Charles Street, and John and Electa would go over what we'd learned that day, while I tried to pay attention. Electa would pull out her laptop, then she and John would write a story of what the doctors had told us, and what the prognosis looked like. Then they'd send an e-mail to other doctors and friends who might know something more about the disease. What we were doing was trying to get a leg up—racing to figure out the best tactic in the fastest way possible. The speed at which things moved was startling.

But sometimes bad news settles slowly. I'm watching the movie on the plane and then deep sounds come from a dry place in my throat I've never felt before. I try to pretend I'm crying over *Atonement* and grab my sweater to hide my tears from Greg Kinnear. Then I stand up to wash my face. It can't be true that there's more cancer. I open a closet door in the plane's galley instead of the bathroom and hear the flight attendant say "She's drunk" to the woman standing near her. But I'm not. Not really. Or maybe a little. I did have the glass of wine after the valium. Or maybe two glasses—it's hard to remember now, and who's counting?

As we drove to the airport for the flight to Boston last week, Lao Wu told Tony he had something he needed to say to me and went on to give a speech in Chinese that had to do with the importance of not worrying. The kids would be fine while I was in Boston, Lao Wu said. I could only catch snippets, so Tony began to translate. Lao Wu said he would make sure the kids were fine. My job was not to worry, he announced as we pulled up to International Departures. My job was to think only good thoughts.

At first, Tony had tried to tell Lao Wu about my cancer and Lao Wu hadn't wanted to hear it. They'd sat in the minivan outside the apartment and Lao Wu put his hands up in the air as if to ward off bad news. He said, "Women bu shi peng you." *We are not friends.* Which was another way of saying they did not have the intimacy needed for such a hard conversation. It seems the Chinese like to talk about sickness and death even less than Americans do.

In the van Tony had to switch tactics with Lao Wu. "Lao Wu," he said. "If we're not friends, then I'm your employer. I pay you to drive the minivan. I need you to know this information about Susan." And this was how Tony got Lao Wu to understand that I had cancer.

Then Lao Wu asked Tony if he believed in Buddhism. Tony told him that he'd read Daoist writings in college and that he was mostly a Daoist. Tony asked Lao Wu what he believed in and Lao Wu said, "The Communist Party doesn't allow anyone to believe." Then he recited a Buddhist poem.

·  ·  ·

We're crossing over the Inner Mongolian plains, an hour or so from Beijing, and I can't stop thinking about the boys. What to say to them? How to say it? In Boston I saw a wise therapist who told me that the best way to talk about breast cancer with children is to tell them the truth. She ran a center for parents with cancer at the hospital. She said we each get one cancer chit to lie to our children with, and that I'd used mine by telling the boys I was at a teaching conference in Boston this week.

The plane lands in the pouring rain and taxis to the gate. A man begins flirting with me at the baggage terminal. He's in his sixties and tells me he's come to China for the car parts industry. I have that feeling again of being on the outside of some great entrepreneurial Chinese gold rush: so many have come from far away to sell plastic bottles and gaskets here. This man says he lived in South America in the 1970s and that it was reckless. I tell him my husband is waiting for me outside customs. He puts his hand on my arm, just for a second, and says he hopes to see me around.

I grab my duffel and find Tony at the gate holding a bouquet of red roses. "They were all I could find," he says, and smiles.

"I feel like we're going to the prom," I joke, and it's good to laugh for a second. Roses are not his style. I'm floating through the terminal. I have so much to tell Tony.

"I'm here," he says quietly while we walk. "I'm here now. Let's sit somewhere. Let's stop."

"But we have to get the kids," I say, looking sideways at him. "Where are the boys?" I remember they're with Hans and Britta—a German couple we met skiing two months ago. They have three kids of their own whom Thorne and Aidan love to play with.

"Britta said to take as long as we want," Tony tells me. "She's planning on giving them dinner."

I'd only known Britta for two months when I called her on the phone ten days ago and told her I was having surgery in Beijing. I didn't want to have to test our new friendship. I didn't want to have to trust it. I sat at my dining room table, and when Britta answered, I said nervously, "We don't know each other well yet, but I'd like to tell someone here that I'm having surgery tomorrow." Britta is a strong woman. She's not easily cowed. That's why I called her.

"I don't want to talk just now," I say to Tony in the newly finished Terminal Three—the largest airport hangar in the world. It's too anonymous in here. "I can't focus on the master plan. I have Thorne and Aidan on the brain."

"We don't need the plan, Sus." Tony takes my arm. "I just need to hear how you are."

"But I want to get the boys," I say. "I need to get them." We walk out under an enormous billboard that reads "My Games, My Contribution, My Happiness." I've seen this sign in Beijing all year. Whose contribution are we talking about, and what kind of happiness?

Back at our apartment Aidan has a drawing of concentric hearts waiting for me. The hearts are in different shades of red magic marker and the word MOMMY is written in blue capital letters in the center. Thorne's made a card out of green construction paper that reads, "I hope you're home for good now."

After I hug the boys and tickle them on the rug in the living room, we sit down at the table to eat bowls of dumplings Tony has warmed up. He wants me to wait to tell the boys until after we've eaten, but I need to get it over with. The hardest part is saying the words out loud: "I have cancer in my breast. My left breast." The boys listen closely. Then Thorne asks me matter-of-factly if I will die. I tell him, "No. I won't die." And it doesn't feel like a lie. It feels like an affirmation.

Aidan asks, "Will you always be okay?" I nod and he seems satisfied. I see that I'm the one with the most fear at the table. The one who's attached meaning to my words. The one with the disease. This is what the Boston therapist also predicted. She told me the boys will want to know if I'm going to live. As long as they know I'm good, then they'll resume their self-focus.

Then Aidan asks me if we know Michelle Obama. He calls her "Michelle" and it takes me a minute to realize whom he's talking about. I laugh and say we don't know Michelle yet.

Thorne wonders, "Does Barack smoke? Because I heard from someone that Barack has tried cigarettes." I say I'm not sure. My face feels flushed. I'm so relieved. Who knew telling the truth could feel so good? The boys' world hasn't stopped with my bad news. They finish their dumplings and ask what's for dessert.

# The Cruelest Month

What happens next is I have to get through the rest of April in China. My breast tissue slides sit in paraffin wax in a pathology lab in western Beijing. I need those slides before we board the plane home. All month long, the head pathologist at the Chinese lab says he's not going to release the slides to me. *It is not their custom*, is how Tony translates what the lab secretary tells him. In China the government has a policy of holding on to everyone's tumor specimens. My breast tissue has become property of the CCCP.

"But they're my wife's," I can hear Tony argue on the phone in English. "It's her tissue. From her body." One week before the flight and Tony switches to Chinese and begins speaking loudly. Our hope is to get the head of the hospital where I had the surgery to call in a favor. I need those slides. They're going to tell the story of my cancer when they're read by pathologists in the States. Meanwhile, I'm killing time in Beijing. I can't concentrate on writing. What if the cancer has slipped into my bloodstream? Or is circulating in my lymphatic system? April is now also the longest month.

There's not much Beijing TV that isn't in Mandarin, and right now I need to be distracted from myself. We have six foreign channels at the apartment. Not bad for a country with no international television ten years ago. But after eight months of the Discovery Channel and National Geographic, I'd love something with a plot. I head out in the van with Lao Wu to an illegal DVD store. I get to a small, nondescript shopping plaza and see a hand-drawn sign: "Tom's Shop." I follow the arrow inside the glass door and take a steep set of spiral stairs that ends in a dank basement where a throng of people rub shoulders among thousands of pirated movies.

A Chinese man I know named Paul cherry-picks American films to air directly on Chinese television. Paul says it's a difficult thing to navigate Chinese censorship. The rules are arbitrary. He told me once at dinner: "You can show boobs, but not nipples." And you can show violence, loads of it, but not against the Chinese government. He says people in China believe concrete rules govern the censoring, and that these rules are written down somewhere. But he's come to realize that the rules are always in a state of flux—like almost everything in this country—made up as the screeners go along.

I'm getting ready to pay for the second season of *Weeds* when one of the teenage girls stocking the shelves runs to the front door, slams it shut, and throws the dead bolt. We're locked in, and from the jittery Mandarin around me it sounds like the police are about to make a raid. The Chinese woman behind the counter starts taking money and selling DVDs fast, then pointing with her hand to the back of the store. I get one huge shot of adrenaline. The police are coming, and they will arrest me and put me in a paddy wagon and take me to jail. I will not be able to speak enough Chinese to make a phone call. I will never see my children again. I won't be able to have the mastectomy.

Why haven't I studied my Chinese harder? I calm down enough to ask clearly, in English, if there is a back door to the store. Another one of the young girls leads me through the stockroom. It's packed with illegal movies—thousands of them in black cases stacked against the wall and in heaps on the floor. I find a secret back staircase, where I run into a line of ten other people standing on steps that lead to a fake door that looks like a wall. I can hear the girl at the top asking quietly for someone on the other side to open up. I finally motion to her to bang on the door—I raise my fist in the air and smile. And so she does, and slowly the wall begins to slide to the side. We are let into an Impressionist art gallery, and from there we fan into the street.

I still have tinglings of the adrenaline when I walk into Jenny Lou's next door to see if they've gotten a shipment of Honey Nut Cheerios. Sometimes they have them, sometimes they don't. Aidan is obsessed with this cereal. It must be a reminder of home for him. Today there are three family-size boxes, and I carry them to the cash register and pay ten dollars for each. The stolen DVDs are a dollar apiece, but the cereal costs five times more than the average Chinese daily wage.

I head back to the minivan and ask Lao Wu if he knows the Chinese word for kung fu. He has no idea what I'm talking about. I want to take the boys to see some kung fu, I say again in my best Mandarin. Finally, I make karate-style air chops, and he gets it right away. He lets out a small yell of recognition. "GONG fu," he says. "Gong fu." The highway is fast today; a whole line of cars is speeding in the breakdown lane as if we're in a NASCAR race. Beeping seems to be the Chinese answer for an indication light.

Then the five lanes are pressed into two with no warning. Cars swerve to avoid hitting a teenage policeman who stands in the middle of the highway wearing a neon orange safety vest. He looks about fifteen and waves a white baton in the air hoping the cars in the road race will see him. I let out a little yell. "Bu keyi." *Not okay.* Lao Wu agrees with me by nodding his head. It's clear he can't speak because the driving has gotten too intense. Cars cut us off and squeal. Up ahead, there's another policeman, just as young as the first, and then another. Where are these boys' mothers?

This is how the highway north of Beijing is cleared of three lanes of traffic for whole miles—by a string of human targets. Just then the first double-decker bus roars past our minivan. Then the second and the third. I begin to piece it together. Only the most important VIPs get the highway cleared for them, and the leaders of the Chinese Communist Party are meeting in Beijing this week. That's them. Stewards of the world's biggest Communist nation speeding by. Maybe I should ask Lao Wu to follow the buses so I can stage a protest. I want these leaders to pass a law allowing pathology labs to release breast tissue of expatriates. "Government?" I ask Lao Wu in English. He nods and tells me in Chinese that the leaders are driving to Tiananmen.

The next day there is good news: Lao Wu takes me to the Chinese lab, where he signs sheafs of forms in triplicate and waits for an orderly to give him my slides. I sit outside the hospital and nervously count the minutes it takes Lao Wu to walk back to the parking lot, open the passenger door, and hand me a box the size of a deck of cards wrapped in a paper towel. This after a month of wrangling.

We drive home to Park Avenue, and I carry the box up to the apartment with two hands—carefully, carefully, as if it's a bird's egg that might break. I put the box in my top bureau drawer, then head back to the elevator. I need to buy milk and bread at the French grocery store before the boys get off the school bus. I run into a Chinese woman I know named Dawn in front of the baskets of oranges. We met on the playground last month, and Dawn told me she was born and raised in Ireland. Her parents emigrated there from China in the sixties simply because they wanted to. She said she's known more discrimination in Beijing than she ever did in Ireland because she can't speak Mandarin. Her English is laced with a beautiful Irish brogue.

She says her mother is in town now. They've just had a family portrait taken. This is when I have an out-of-body experience in the produce section and tell Dawn I've got breast cancer. I must need to unload, because I don't know Dawn well enough for this. But here I am, bursting with news. Dawn's advice: *Eat organic. Eat only organic.* She says, *You have to. And no stress. You can't have any stress.* I nod my head and want to laugh. There's one week left until my mastectomy and she thinks everything will be okay if I can just get my hands on some organic Chinese produce.

Tonight Britta brings us dinner. She and Hans and Tony and I sit at our dining table and try not to talk about cancer. She and Hans are from Germany by way of London and have been in China for two years. When I met Britta, my dating circle widened dramatically. She invited me to book clubs and brunches and craft fairs. She's a milliner by trade and designs great hats for women all over the world.

Hans passes the plate of cheeses to me and asks Tony how he learned Chinese. "It's a story of chance," Tony says. "I stood in the hall of the language department at Stanford twenty-four years ago thinking I'd sign up for Japanese. There was a long line outside that office. Everyone wanted to learn Japanese then. A Chinese teacher offered me a cup of tea. There was no one in the Chinese line. When I left, I had registered for beginning Mandarin."

Hans laughs. "I think knowing the language makes all the difference here."

"It certainly helps." Tony nods.

"And I believe," Hans adds, taking a sip of red wine, "you're either outside the language or inside the language in China. What I mean is, you're either in the conversation or not in it." He stops and smiles. "So you are in." He points at Tony. Then he looks over to Britta and me. "And we are out."

I try to pay attention, but I can't. What I want is for someone to tell me that the pain in my side is a bruised rib or perhaps a pulled muscle. I'm struggling. Britta and Hans are sincere. It's good to have them here. I am so glad we met them. I don't have to try to laugh with them. If the cancer has already changed me in any way, it's that I'm more honest. This is a good thing. I can also now detect bullshit from a mile away.

In the morning, Sabrina and I take our four children horseback riding for the first time, deep into the dry forest north of Beijing. Lao Wu drives us forty-five minutes on the crowded highway until we near the airport, where I can see the planes coming down low. Then we veer off the road into the woods. Sabrina leans forward and tells me there's some übersurgeon who "does breasts" at a Beijing public hospital, but you have to wait years to see him, unless you know someone who can grease the wheels. She asks me if I would like her to try to arrange an appointment with him. "No," I say. "No thank you."

Then she asks, "Are you feeling tired today?" I know this is the indirect Chinese way of saying she's thinking about my cancer. I'm grateful. But I'm also afraid. I don't want to have to trust my new friendships here. I'm worried that these women won't meet me halfway. Or won't be able to. Introducing cancer into new courtships is not very Jane Austen. I'm sure it's frowned upon in etiquette books.

Sabrina wonders if I want to ride a horse and I shake my head. Three old men in black wool jackets sit by the side of the road smoking cigarettes. One blue dump truck full of wooden beams stops in the middle and forces us to drive around it. There are no other cars. I want to tell Sabrina that I'm certain cancer has infiltrated my bones. I could not be more serious. My left arm hurts, so I try not to move it. I don't want to disturb tumors growing there. All this anxiety has given me a stomachache.

We come upon a couple of half-formed cinder-block foundations and then rows of poplar trees that line the banks of a slow green river. The land seems to have been untouched for centuries, even this close to the capital. Tony would say I'm imagining things with my arm. Last night he called Dr. Specht, my wonderful surgeon back in the States, who said that under no circumstances would my small cancer be causing my arm to hurt and that what I was feeling was radial pain from the lumpectomies. Dr. Specht said, "Try to get her to sleep."

Then we come upon the surprise of the Sheerwood horse farm—a sprawling compound of riding rings and aluminum barns with hundreds of stalls tucked in the forest like in a fairy tale. The children jump out of the van and run to try on riding helmets. Then they each climb up on a horse and spend an hour learning how to post, while I stand in the eighty-degree heat watching and feeling deranged. I try not to think about my cancer for minutes at a time. Sabrina comes and stands beside me and says, "Thorne is a natural on the horse. And look at Aidan. Look at how he talks to his pony."

Thorne is on a gigantic black mare that holds her head

high while he rides her in circles in the ring. He smiles and smiles and waves to me. Aidan is in the fenced-in ring on a white pony that bucks. But Aidan murmurs to him and shows him how to be friends. My mind is like a gerbil on an exercise wheel. It circles the cancer over and over. Can my children sense how tense I am? All I want to do is get to Boston and have the surgery. I'm not prepared for anything that might come after—not dying, or talking to my kids more about dying. I'm not prepared to feel mortal.

After the boys fall asleep that night, Tony and I try to watch an old James Bond movie on TV. It's an odd thing to look at Sean Connery speaking Mandarin. I lean back on the couch, and Tony rubs my feet. Then I run my hand along my elbow and find a lump under the skin. It's been there for years, but I turn to Tony and hold my arm out.

"Look," I say. Proof of the cancer.

"It's nothing, Sus," he says calmly. "You've always had that bump. It's from where your elbow rubs against the edge of the desk when you write." Then he stands and puts his hand out to walk me to the bedroom. "Let's go to sleep." Tony's love holds us up right now. But I miss my friends. I miss my family. It's time to go home.

The plan is to take the boys out of school on Friday, eight weeks before the semester ends, and move in with my parents in Maine. We'll land there on a Wednesday and then two days later Tony and I will drive to Boston for my surgery. Who knows when we'll come back to China? Or if we will. We have to pack as if we're gone for good.

But before we go we need to orchestrate a series of good-byes—to Rose, to my yoga teacher, Mimi. To the boys' school. We need to make this leave-taking feel within the realm of normal. I worry that pulling Thorne and Aidan from school is too big a disruption, but Julie, the school principal and also my friend, reminds me how resilient children are. She tells me the teachers are putting together a road packet for the time the boys will miss. She convinces me that Thorne and Aidan will love going home for summer early.

We finally arrive at the "day before we're leaving China." I didn't think I'd reach it. There's been this urgency following me. A dark feeling I can't shake. At the bus stop in the morning, two of the Taiwanese moms give me farewell cards with short Bible verses inscribed in them. My friend Flora hugs me and says "I love you" into my ear. All along, there have been limits to these playground friendships. But Flora says "I love you," and for just one moment I believe her. It's one of those lost-in-translation moments; Flora does not really love me. She doesn't even know me well. What I think she means to say is that she sends her love, or wishes me well. It's freakishly warm—seventy-five degrees in April—but the desert wind is in our faces, and I notice that Flora and I are still wearing parkas to stay warm.

In the afternoon I go to Mimi's apartment and we do yoga poses to try to loosen my arm on the surgery side. She says the pain I'm having there is a pressed nerve, not cancer. She has me lie on a bolster and stretches my torso until the pressure begins to release. I stay on the floor with my eyes closed. She says, "Try repeating these words: 'I open to what is.'"

I make my mind quiet and then I begin. I say *I open to what is* to myself and the phrase feels vaguely powerful. I say it again. It sounds familiar, even. Like I've been waiting to say it. *I open to what is.* Somehow repeating these simple words begins to unlock the box for me. Some of the tension is let out.

# IV

# Palace of Tranquil Longevity

# 交泰殿

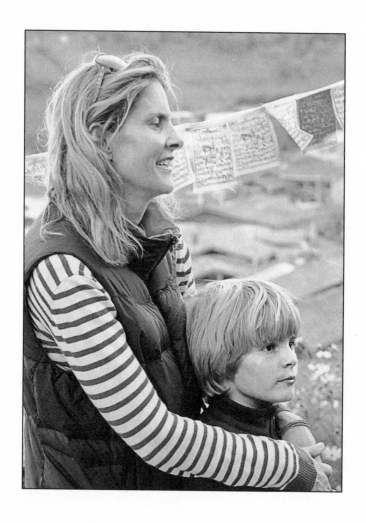

Susan and Thorne resting outside of Shangri-La in the Deqen Tibetan Autonomus region of Yunnan Province

# Clouds or Butterflies

Cancer follows us to Maine and up to the second floor of the old wooden house that my parents have given over to us. I think my mother has made some vow I'll never know about to not cry in front of me. Around me she's steady and calm. Crying used to be one of my mother's clear forms of expression— one of her gifts. Something you could count on, because happy or sad, my mother would cry. But I can't be around crying right now. This is why I know there's been some vow. Because she doesn't cry. She doesn't tell me how terrible all this is. She just helps me.

My sister, Erin, has flown in from San Francisco for the week. She's the fun aunt who does art projects with maple leaves and glue at the dining room table, then plays rock music during dinner and gets the boys to eat their green beans. The mastectomy is scheduled for tomorrow at noon in Boston. Tony will drive us down today after lunch. My friend Lily will fly in from Italy, where she and her two girls and her husband are living in a village north of Florence for the year. She sends Tony an e-mail with her flight number and jokes that it will be a relief to leave the freak rains that have drenched most of Italy that month. But Lily doesn't like to fly, and the fact that she's already in the air, making her way to me in Boston, turns the surgery into something real. Something I can get through.

Aidan finds me in the kitchen and hands me a drawing he's made on pink construction paper. He's all business. "Mommy. When you have the surgery, you should keep this drawing near you."

There are thirty or so pink and purple butterflies under a bed of blue clouds. The wings of each butterfly have been carefully drawn to look like the butterflies are in midflight. "It's so pretty, Aidan," I say. "It must have taken a lot of work."

We have to be at Massachusetts General Hospital at eight the next morning for pre-op. The surgery won't start until about ten. Aidan says, "You have to choose which one you want to be during your surgery—clouds or butterflies." He looks up at me, waiting, and I realize he's offering me a way to escape the operating room. How does he know I need this? How has he gotten it so right?

"Which do you want to be?"

"Butterfly," I decide almost without thinking. "I want to be a butterfly."

"Okay." He nods and smiles slightly, like I've made a good choice. He stares at the drawing for a minute longer and then points. "Now you can imagine you're one of these butterflies in this drawing if the surgery hurts." He pauses again. "Which butterfly do you think is the prettiest? You've got to pick one."

There are so many beautiful butterflies it's almost impossible to choose, but I point to one. "Okay." He nods again and seems to approve. "Okay. Now this is your butterfly." He stares at me briefly, right in the eyes. "Imagine you're this butterfly during the surgery, okay? Then, whenever you want, you can just fly away." He says the last part slowly, like he's giving me the keys to the universe. Then he adds, "You just get up and fly away." He looks at me for another second, to make sure I've got it, then heads to the backyard to play a game of Wiffle ball with my father and Erin and Thorne, who are waiting for him.

When I wake up after the surgery, I seem to be in a hospital bed in Boston overlooking the Charles River. I can tell I'm talking a lot; too much, probably. Lily and Electa and Tony have stopped answering, and they stare at me from the little red couch by the window. I babble about how good I feel and ask if they think I'll be able to get up soon and take a shower. I wonder when we can have lunch. Tony says slowly, "You seem really good, Sus. I'm surprised by how good you seem." Then I get up from the bed to go wash my face, dragging my IV pole behind me. My friend Genevieve has sent me an incredible care package with chocolates and hand cream and Swedish fish. I lie back in bed and ask Tony where the candy is.

Dr. Specht comes to check on me and I tell her I can hardly feel the pain. "That's the morphine talking." Dr. Specht laughs and checks my chart. "You're all about the painkillers right now."

After she leaves, Lily stands up from the couch and hands me a blank writing book with a pale blue cover. "It's something I got in Italy," she says. "Maybe for you to write in." I look at her like she's crazy. Because there's nothing to write about here. Nothing worth remembering. I want to tell her I won't be chronicling this disease. I will be forgetting the IV and the morphine and the view to the river as soon as I leave this blue hospital room.

"Just in case," she adds. "Because writing might help. Writing might be a way to get through this." I smile at her and put the book on the table next to the bed. I don't want to see it again.

When the morphine wears off, the nurse gives me Percocet, which always makes me throw up, and so I do, into a bedpan Tony holds next to the bed. Then quickly the Charles River does not look as sparkling. The Boston sky seems grayer. I become quieter and take a long nap. In the morning Electa drives us to a nearby hotel, and we camp out there for two days: me and Tony and Lily and Electa and Electa's husband, Jos, who is one of Tony's best friends and who comes and goes, bringing take-out food. On the second night, they eat Indian curries in their laps and we watch a film on Lily's computer about two lonely musicians in Prague who almost get together and then don't. I am not hungry. The sound track is haunting, and I find the movie unbearably sad. I lie on the couch riding out the pain, and the film seems to be about death in the end—loneliness and death. Everyone else in the hotel room enjoys the movie, and it scares me to feel so disconnected from these people I love. I kick the Percocet in the morning. I kick all the painkillers. They're not doing me any good. And I begin, right away, to feel more pain, but also a lot more like myself.

Now if I lie very still in my old spool bed, with my left arm propped up on a stack of pillows, I can keep the pain from spreading down my ribs. It feels like someone has burrowed a knife into my chest and armpit. The boys have gone to sleep in their beds after snuggling with me while Tony read them a chapter from *The Wind in the Willows*. He and I hold hands and watch TV news. There was a large earthquake in China two days after we left Beijing. The reports today say that over fifty thousand people have died in Sichuan Province. Tony says

Tibetans live in that region, and he thinks the Chinese will see the earthquake as retribution for Tibetan protests this spring.

The next report is about a cyclone in Burma that has killed thousands. The footage shows flooded Burmese villages. Then the story switches back to the fallen-down schools near Chengdu, in central China. I can see parents weeping in the background and others walking the perimeter of heaps of rubble in a daze. It's a terrible thing to watch—these people in so much private suffering. I close my eyes and wonder what Lao Wu is hearing about the earthquake. He does not have a television. He gets his news from Chinese radio. I hope he doesn't have family in Sichuan.

Tony finally turns off the TV. I lie in the dark and stare at the ceiling. Tony falls asleep next to me, and I finger the drainage pipe under the sheets—it's a piece of thin, plastic tubing that comes out of my skin somewhere near the middle of my rib cage. It transfers pinkish fluid from my surgery site into a small plastic bag that hangs off the corset the doctors have fastened me into. We need to get the pipe out soon.

I'm struck then by how cancer is itself a kind of cultural dislocation. I feel more removed from myself—more distanced now from the people I love than I ever did in China. And why all this sadness? My left breast is gone, and the surgeon has replaced it with a silicone implant, which is vaguely unsettling. All I feel there now is numbness. My hope is that the surgeon did all she could do. I hope she got the cancer out.

During the next week friends come. I sit on my mother's couch and try to take in the faces of these women I love. I've missed them these last nine months in China. But now sometimes my connection to them feels fleeting. I see them, but I can't really hear them. It's as if the cancer has somehow separated me from them. I'm astonished at how much work it is to try to talk. I nod my head. I smile. But I'm not even me anymore. I'm someone different—someone with this loss. I just can't explain it yet.

Sometimes I'm distracted now around the boys. Detached. I can't quite get my hands on them—I can't hug them yet because of the tube and the plastic drainage bag, and I can't move my left arm because of the pain. I don't feel entirely like their person anymore. Maybe I'm a different version of myself—a woman with a fake left breast pretending to be their mother. And I have to give a lot of the parenting up to the group. While I was in the hospital, the boys took to the game of Wiffle ball with even more ferocity. Now they spend hours batting and pitching with imaginary base runners and outfielders. There are so many friends who take Thorne and Aidan away for swimming and pizza and ice cream. Tony's brother, Peter, keeps shuttling the boys to the YMCA to shoot hoops. I can't think too much about the distance between the boys and me right now or it makes me sad.

Tuesday marks one week since my mastectomy, and I walk downtown to buy flaxseed at the health food store in Bath. I've read that it helps stave off cancer. I'm busy now looking for a cure. For an elixir. I'm trying to keep the sadness at bay. The walk takes ten minutes and it's my longest since the surgery. People go in and out of the local bank and Wilson's Drugstore, but there's no larger white noise here, just the sound of wind and the river down below.

Beijing was so loud—the crashing of bulldozers and cranes and the screeching of truck brakes. I pass a woman I recognize on the sidewalk, the mother of a friend from middle school who says she'd heard I was in China. She asks me if the Chinese people were nice to me. I smile because I never know how to answer this question; it always seems beside the point. I want to say that there are so many other things I could tell her about China.

On Wednesday, my friend Katie flies up from Brooklyn to see me. We take a slow walk down to the river. There's an explosion of tulips and hydrangeas and trellis roses along the way. After lunch in a café, we stand under a lilac tree in my parents' driveway and we talk about cancer and about our love for our children. And it feels like we can talk for days. Then Katie says, "I love the smell of lilacs. It's spring to me."

I smile and say, "Yes. That's it." I am so glad she's come. I'm done talking now. Exhausted. And happy we can sit in the backyard quietly now and watch.

I'm learning that cancer tends to live in a wordless place. On Saturday, a friend of my mother's named Judith arrives. I've been wearing the hospital corset for almost ten days, and it's begun to make grooves and small sores in the skin along my rib cage. Judith has just finished her EMT shift for the Brunswick Fire Department. She has me sit on the couch so she can unzip the front flap of the corset and unpin the plastic tubing and remove the pouch attached to the tubing that holds the pink runoff. Then she begins to rub cream on my skin. She doesn't talk, except to say that the doctors made the corset too tight. It feels good to have the thing off.

I've come to feel as if I'm bobbing in a lake where only people with cancer swim. It's a big lake. My husband is sitting by my side on the floor next to the couch holding the tubing while Judith massages me. But he is not in the lake. Only people with cancer can be in the lake. So where Tony is could best be described as on the shore waiting for me to come back. Maybe he is rummaging in the forest for wood to make a fire to keep us warm. But the biggest surprise of all is still that Tony is not in the lake. That he's never going to be able to swim in the lake. *He doesn't have cancer.* The thin line between having and not having seems malleable sometimes, but for me that line is everything. It separates. I lie on the couch after Judith leaves and hold on to Tony's hand until I feel most of the solitude wash away.

# Decade by Decade

The words *lymph nodes* keep playing in my head. Lymph nodes. Lymph nodes. On Monday the pathology report is in, and Tony and I speed south on I-95. I'm too nervous. Tony has the radio turned up to a story about huge profits in the oil industry. The second story is about the earthquake in China. So is the third. One reporter looks at the psychological effects of the quake. Another examines the crowded refugee camps. The latest statistics say fifty-one thousand are dead. Twenty-nine thousand remain missing. Five million are homeless, and the number is sure to grow. The Chinese government has asked the world to send six million tents.

Tony and the boys and I had been planning to take a train to Chengdu for the spring break in May until we had to leave early. There's a panda preserve north of the city in Wolong that's been destroyed in the quake. Most of the pandas in the world live in this swath of wrecked land in central southern China.

One of the mud flaps on a flatbed truck we pass reads, "Jesus is Lord." The other says, "Driving for God." The fourth radio story takes us back to oil because today the price of one barrel has spiked to $135. We pass a gas station near Kittery with a sign outside: "Worms and crawlers for sale cheap."

I see an old Chrysler sedan up ahead with a large digital photo of Jesus Christ laminated to the back window. "Oh," I say to Tony. "Look at that." The car speeds onto the highway from the right and never yields. The whole time I was in Beijing, I never saw one image of Jesus Christ.

Tony puts on his blinker and moves to the left lane to make room. The picture of Jesus takes up most of the car's back window. "Wouldn't see that in China," he says, reading my mind.

When we get to the hospital, I sit down in the oncologist's office and the first thing Dr. Holland tells me is she hopes I live at least fifty more years. This is her goal for me, she explains, and I think it's a worthy one, but I'm surprised by her candor. It takes me a minute to realize we're talking seriously about how many years I have left to live. I announce I'm entirely on board with her plan. But what I want to say is could we skip this because this part is too depressing.

Then Dr. Holland says we'll solve my health problems "decade by decade." She explains that the pathology shows I have a good chance of being alive in ten years. "That's when your sons will graduate from high school," she says. "That's not so bad, is it? In fact, that's good," she adds.

"It is?" I ask. But the words I want to say are *What language are you speaking?* Is there some piece of the pathology report I've missed? The lymph nodes are clear. Alive to see the boys graduate from high school? I can reach out and touch high school. I want college. I want weddings. Grandchildren. What I learn next is that there was a third tumor hiding in the mastectomy tissue. Dr. Holland puts a good face on it—and almost tricks me into believing her. She says I've gotten a B today instead of an A on the story of my cancer.

I'm sitting in the small, windowless office and Dr. Holland's face begins to spin. This is the sneaky thing cancer does—it displaces me. I believe it's ten in the morning on a Tuesday in Boston, but then I'm cast adrift on some roiling swell of mortality. I close my eyes. Thinking of my kids helps. Last night when I tucked Aidan into bed, he reached for me and announced, "This hug will be for ten minutes."

# Chinese Blessing

Rose has sent me to Maine with a tiny brass charm in a green silk pouch. I carry it with me everywhere. On the small card inside the bag she's written:

> *Susan Conley will be okay!*
> *Susan Conley will be fine!*
> *Susan Conley will be all right!*

It's a Chinese blessing she's translated into English that I'm supposed to keep near me always.

At the bottom of the blessing, she's written:

*Dear Susan,*
   *I'll be here in Beijing, waiting for you to come back and continue your Chinese lessons.*
   *Rose*

# You Are Here

July comes and Tony flies back to China. He writes me an e-mail when he lands in Beijing, remembering our first road trip together, when we drove eighteen hours to Baja for the weekend. We camped in the desert on a futon mattress we pulled from the back of the truck. I woke up in the sand on the first night and looked at millions of tiny stars in the sky. "Tony," I said and grabbed his arm while he slept. I hardly knew him. But I also already knew him entirely. "Tony, where are we?"

He sat up too and stared at the Mexican sky and said slowly, "I don't know where we are." Then we both lay down and put our arms around each other and went back to sleep.

The next week Tony cooked Chinese noodles in his rented house in San Francisco. He loved to make dinner for crowds in his big, iron wok. He still does. That night he wore a long-sleeved blue T-shirt that had the solar system printed on it in white. The words "You Are Here" were written next to planet Earth with a small arrow. He'd worn the T-shirt to give me the answer I'd needed back in Baja. *You Are Here.* He turned to me from where he stood at the stove and smiled his calm smile, and I swear that night was when I knew I would marry him.

. . .

After Tony leaves, the boys and I move out of town to an old cottage that our family's had for thirty years. There's room for all of us—my parents; my sister, Erin, who comes again in August to help; my brother, John, his wife, Jenna, and their sweet baby, Lyla. This place used to be a boys' camp in the 1800s, and the names of the campers—William St. John, Ezra Sturm, Henry Keyes—are still carved in the walls of the upstairs bedrooms.

I drive into town every day for radiation, but mostly I lie on the couch and look at the ocean. More than anything, I have missed seeing this body of water. I like to watch it change moods. The ocean to me suggests greatness. It suggests pre-historic whales and huge expanses of time. There are lobster traps out in front, and the same tall, spindly blue heron stands in the cove on one foot. You can pick blueberries from the bush while you walk to the car.

This morning the boys eat Cheerios while we look out at a big fog. The air is thick and reminds me of the worst smog in Beijing. *The Sound of Music* plays on the CD player, and Thorne sings along to every word of "Do-Re-Mi."

"Stop, Thorne," Aidan says. "Too loud." He's working hard on a drawing of a sheep.

"Why don't you just listen to the music," I suggest to Thorne. Then he announces out of nowhere that he's mad at me because I'm already forty.

"I wish you were only thirty," Thorne says with a serious face. I put down the article I'm reading about vitamins I need to boost my immune system. "You're forty," Thorne says again. "So that means you only have forty more years to live."

*If you only knew,* I want to say to him. *If you only had any idea of how hard I'm working to pull off the next ten.* "But I'm going to live until I'm one hundred," I say, and smile at him, half believing myself.

"You are?" He smiles back. "Can you live until two hundred?"

I say, "Only a certain kind of tortoise from the Galápagos Islands can." Then Aidan puts down his sheep drawing and stands up with a dreamy look on his face. Do these boys know what I would do for them? Now that the tubing is out and the corset is off, my love for them is more accessible. I do not need as much distance from them. I don't need to take as many breaks in the room inside my head.

"Mom." Aidan stares at me intently. "Are there invisible people who can go in and out of our bodies like the wind?"

I look him in the eye and say back equally seriously, "Aidan. I just don't know."

Then Tony calls to report that the pollution was so bad on Monday in Beijing he couldn't see the Rem Koolhaas CCTV Tower from our bedroom window. It's the new landmark skyscraper everyone is buzzing about, and on good air days it seems to be very close to our apartment. On bad air days the smog makes everything shrouded and you wonder what everyone's doing huddled together in a chemical soup out in the middle of the desert.

Tony explains that the government seeded the clouds for the Olympics. "They what?" I ask.

"They fabricated a rainstorm. Seeded the clouds. Shot chemical pellets up into the sky until it rained and washed the smog away."

"You're kidding."

"No. And last night at the opening ceremony in the Bird's Nest the sky was clear. Clear." He says there were more people onstage and more energy in that stadium than I could ever imagine watching on TV. Now he's just gotten back from beach volleyball in the park across from our apartment. "The whole concession stand concept does not seem to translate here," he says. "I was at the volleyball for five hours and all they had for sale was warm beer."

"We looked for you on TV," I tell him. "The boys cannot get over the fact that it's Beijing on the screen. They keep begging to watch more."

After we each say good-bye, the boys and I make our way to the beach. In the car, Aidan asks, "Mom, who made the first tree?"

I take a breath. I think I can tell where this conversation is going. "Remember how I told you different people believe different things? Some people think a god made the first tree. Some people believe in the science that made cells that grew into plants like the very first tree."

"A tree god." Aidan smiles. He's already alchemized my words into something he can hold on to. "Maybe there's a tree god." What a good idea that would be.

"Yeah," Thorne adds. "A tree god would be great!"

"But maybe"—Aidan gets serious now again—"we'll never know for sure. Do you think we'll ever know, Mom?"

Aidan is asking me about the mystery of the universe on Tuesday at eleven in the morning on the way to Popham Beach, and I want to be honest with him. It's my new cancer policy. "Probably not, Aidan," I say. "We will probably never know for absolute sure who made the first tree."

"But, Mom," he says, calmly now, "if you're out somewhere and you learn the answer—like if somebody tells you who made the universe—will you come home and tell me?"

"Tell both of us!" Thorne yells. "Make sure you tell us both!"

"I will," I say, looking in the rearview mirror. "I will make sure I do that."

. . .

After we've come back from the beach and gotten the sand off our feet with the hose and eaten our hot dogs, it's bedtime. The lights are out in the boys' room, but the sun has just set and the orange glow comes through the curtains. I tuck Thorne in. "Are you strong?" he asks me from his bed. "Let me see your biceps." He's begun to be interested in people's strength—in how physically big they are. "Let me see," Thorne demands.

Aidan's eyes are closed. I'm tired tonight and want to go to sleep right after the boys do. I'm missing Tony. I flex my arms and show Thorne my small muscles. "You're strong," he decides and sounds surprised. Then he looks me in the eye and asks me clearly, "Are you strong enough to survive?"

*Whoa,* I think. *I didn't see that one coming.*

"Yes," I say. I feel like Thorne is willing me to live. Like he knows what the stakes are. Like he's known all along. I look at him and I don't flinch. "Yes," I say again, "I'm strong enough." Then I kiss him on the cheek and close his door and go lie down on the floor in my bedroom until I feel like I've stopped shaking and can stand up.

# Spaceship

Last Tuesday, the day it poured rain, I drove to New Hampshire to see a traditional Chinese medicine doctor friends had told me about. Dr. Wang had a poster on the wall of the human body with the meridian points written in Chinese. She told me that after the Cultural Revolution, she was able to get out of China and eventually make it to the States. She asked me a lot of quick questions that implied she already knew the answers: "Do you get stressed often?" "Do you worry?" I'd heard this stuff before—the idea that women like me go too fast. Work too hard. That we cause our own cancers. It's a dangerous brand of reasoning. "You must have been very run-down in the years both your boys were babies at the same time," Dr. Wang said next.

"No more than any other woman," I answered. "And I'm really not that stressed." I decided I wasn't going to make the consultation so easy for her. I wanted to tell Dr. Wang that in my house we have family meals. Play board games. I'm a freelance writer and teacher, not a corporate executive. How much stress can there be?

That was when Dr. Wang said, "Something in your life caused your immune system to fail." *Oh, please,* I wanted to say with my voice raised. *Oh, come on.*

All of this suggested that my cancer was my own doing, and that I had not, to quote Dr. Wang, been cultivating enough chi. I was also apparently drinking too many cold beverages. "Too much ice," she told me. "Did you know ice is bad for chi?" All my life I have searched out ice cubes, even if it meant poking around in other people's crowded freezers.

"No, I didn't know that," I said and closed my eyes, trying to figure out how quickly I could get out of there.

Today my mother and I finally take the boys to the cancer center in Bath to see the radiation machine. We pass the Community Gun Club—a sagging green wooden shed off Route 209 with a sign out front that reads "Trapping Course. August 13–17. Talk to Dan."

We pass the old rec center and my junior high school. "Just bring the kids in for a peek," Dr. Godin had said last week. "That way they won't think what you're doing is so scary." She's the radiation oncologist in charge of my daily dose. She's a cool customer and one of the most inspiring doctors on the whole team. The day I met her she looked me in the eye and said, *We have one chance to get this radiation thing right and then you go live your life.*

So here, at the halfway point in my treatment, my boys run through the front door of the center ahead of my mother and me. I poke my head down the nurses' hall and see Rachel, one of the fabulous technicians. "The boys are here," I say. "Is that okay?"

"Of course it's okay." She smiles. "I'll be ready for you in five and we'll bring them in."

I will now admit that I find getting daily radiation comforting. It's inconvenient and dehumanizing and sometimes I cry on the table for no reason. But at least I know I'm being *treated*. I've decided that more than anything cancer is a simple game of biological luck. I want as much luck on my side as I can garner, plus all the radiation the doctors will give me.

Which will turn out to be exactly thirty-one days of it. The boys won't sit down in the waiting room. My mother stands in the open doorway trying to corral them. They keep hovering close to study the long cotton johnny I've thrown on. This one is covered in small blue flowers. "What is that thing you're wearing, Mommy?" Thorne asks and reaches out to touch my wide sleeve. "It's weird-looking. It's for sick people."

There's one other man in the room with us. He looks to be in his seventies and has belted a blue cotton bathrobe over his striped johnny. He reads the newspaper, and even though he's smiled at me many times before, and together we've guessed if it will ever rain this August, he never once looks over the top of his paper the whole time the boys are in the room. I decide it just isn't possible for him today—that we all have days when we feel the cancer is beating us, and maybe this is one of his days.

There are too many things for the boys to finger in the waiting room: stacks of slippery magazines and a small plastic globe, pull cords on the roman shades. The boys are excited—it's a hot day, and we're going to the beach after this. They begin a game of tag down the carpeted hall toward the nurses' station, until my mother grabs one of their hands and stops them. *What are they doing here?* I want to ask someone. Because they look so out of place. Maybe this was a bad idea, bringing them.

Then Aidan decides to do yoga in the waiting room. "This is a sun salutation," he announces and lies down in the middle of the rug. Which is when Rachel pops her head in and asks us if we're ready. The boys run to her, and she leads us into the radiation room, which is always surprisingly cold (the computers, I've been told, like it cold) and loud. We have to scream-talk while we explain the TomoTherapy machine to the boys. They stare at it silently like it's some kind of spaceship.

Thorne doesn't say much in the room. I know he's taking it all in. He looks quickly at me where I stand next to the bed and then at his grandmother expectantly. I decide that when you are five or seven, a visit to your mom's radiation room is meant to be short. "Wow" is all Aidan says.

My mother takes both boys by the hands and says, "Bye-bye, Mommy. We'll see you out in the car." And I smile at them and hold back my tears. I'm thankful for my mother again—for how she knows what needs to happen.

"Wow," Aidan repeats while they walk toward the door. "That machine is really big." I'm still not sure if bringing them in was a mistake. I do know that neither of the boys has ever mentioned one thing about the radiation center to me since.

# V

# Palace of Earthly Tranquility

# 交泰殿

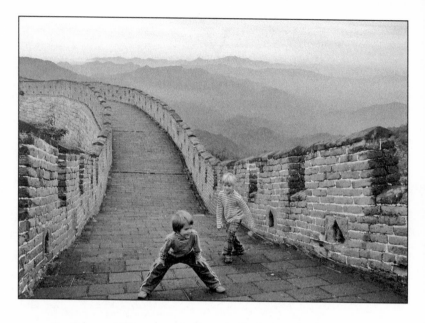

Aidan and Thorne on the Great Wall of China at Mutianyu

# How to Hire an Ayi

In the middle of August Tony flies back to Maine and packs us up, and then the four of us board the return flight to Beijing. We land a little after three on a Thursday, and all of us seem to have slept during the night; except Tony, who for some reason decided he needed to watch *Taxi Driver,* one of the darkest movies ever. We deplane and he's catatonic. We have a lot of bags. Twelve, I think. Each one of us has to push a metal cart stacked with them. We wheel our load to the customs line, where they take each bag and scan it. Tony's cart is stacked the highest, and every bag of his falls off in a pile on the floor as we reach the head of the line. I try hard not to laugh. It's hot in the terminal, and once again, I'm not sure where we are.

If I'm not careful, China could become an adversary. Because I've arrived looking for evidence that we shouldn't have returned: the toxic air. The traffic. The spitting. If you want reasons to flee Beijing, they abound. We make it out into the teeming terminal and need to find an elevator up to the floor where Lao Wu waits. But I can't get my cart to turn around. Its wheels won't budge. Then the whole thing tips and I almost lose the bags. The boys and Tony are on the elevator calling for me, but I'm still in the main thoroughfare—an American woman with ratty hair trying to dodge people and yank the cart around, but I can't manage it. Finally a teenage guard pops up from a line of guards sitting in chairs watching. He never laughs at me, which I think is noble, and he turns me around and gets me on my way.

We drive back to the apartment and I dig in my bags for a book of Maine photos I've brought for Lao Wu. I smile when I give it to him. We've missed him so much. And then we shake hands because I've learned it's too embarrassing for him if we hug. Inside the apartment it looks like we've just returned from breakfast. This is a comforting feeling, but also disorienting. How long have we been away? A week? A month? A year? Long enough for me to have cancer? Have I really had two surgeries? Have I been lying under that radiation machine every day for the last six weeks? Where did the time go? And that breast? And that sickening fear?

Xiao Wang is waiting for us at the door. I give her an embrace, awkward because of the hugging question. On the whole, China has not seemed like a hugging nation to me. There's a great deal more talking here than hugging. But I'm happy to see Xiao Wang, so I can't stop myself, and I reach for her tiny torso and squeeze it, and she half squeezes me back. I ask her about her son and she says he's still much better. "No IV," she tells me in English. "No more crying." Then she grabs the duffels off the elevator and helps me haul them into the front hall. She's serious about unpacking. She pulls one of the bigger bags into our bedroom and within minutes she's cornered Tony in there and is fast talking about how she's quitting. He translates for me as I pass by on my way to see how many of the plants have survived (just one) and I think he must be kidding. She's what? She's kidding. We paid her all summer while we've been gone.

At first, Xiao Wang says she'll only be gone a month or so. Her husband has to go back to their province and pack up his elderly grandfather and grandmother, who've lost their house to the earthquake. Now who will watch her son? These are serious times in China after the earthquake. But we'll wait for her return, I tell her. I also want to say I'm sure we can work out a schedule that suits her, but I can't manage these subordinate clauses in Mandarin.

My Chinese has vanished. Gone. I think I lost it somewhere around the third week of radiation. I wonder if it will ever return. Xiao Wang says she has a friend who lives in her village, Mao Ayi, who will work for us for the month. It's all been planned. We've been back in China a little more than two hours. I nod while Xiao Wang announces that she'll bring Mao Ayi with her to the apartment tomorrow so we can meet her. *You will like her,* she commands us. Tony gets quiet and translates less and less of what Xiao Wang is saying. I can tell it's gotten serious. My arm and rib cage are tight and stiff from the radiation and the long flight. I need to stretch them out. I wish Xiao Wang would leave the bedroom so I could lie down on the floor. This is when she adds that her husband has decided that the bus commute is too long for her. What's worse, she gets bus sick. Once she fainted on the bus last spring and had to go straight to the hospital.

She's refolding my underwear and bras and placing them in small piles on the rug. This is uncomfortable because I could do this part. I can fold underwear. There are other, magical things Xiao Wang does that I can't do: like speak Chinese to the maintenance men when the water mysteriously goes off, and play badminton in the hall with the boys. Soon it's clear that Xiao Wang is going away for a lot longer than a month. She plans to receive her month's salary today and take that bus ride home.

Then she admits that she's a terrible cook. She hates to cook, she says. Tony translates each sentence, and I have to turn away to stop from smiling. She confesses that she'd never really cooked a meal before she began working for us. Her husband is the cook. Each day last year she phoned him and he dictated recipes. She tells Tony she doesn't like to handle the meat. This explains why the food she made us was so often a glop that all of us had a hard time eating. And why it was almost always shaved pork in oil or shaved chicken in oil. Lots of oil. We felt bad about the food Xiao Wang cooked. It was a wonderful thing to have someone in my kitchen making dinner. But I felt guilty that we couldn't eat the meals Xiao Wang made, and I felt guilty about complaining, because how many people are lucky enough to have someone actually cooking for them. What a treat.

It became a routine: the boys would push the chicken in oil or pork in oil around their plate with their wooden chopsticks, and after ten minutes or so, I'd pour out the Honey Nut Cheerios. But I was so grateful for Xiao Wang—she understood how to work the washing machine. She helped me order the drinking water. She sang Chinese songs to help the boys go to sleep on the nights she stayed late. Now Xiao Wang finishes unpacking our bags and goes home. We have been back in the country just over five hours. Tony hustles to the computer and finds three unemployed ayis on a Web site. I'm impressed. He's showing verve. He's worried we won't hit it off with Xiao Wang's friend. He's learned she doesn't speak a single word of English, and I agree this could be a problem.

I stand in the living room, staring at the moving cars on the Fourth Ring Road. I feel deceived by the air pollution. It's just as bad as the day I left in May. I feel deceived by Xiao Wang, though I know I can't really blame her. I decide I've been deceived firstly and mostly by NBC, because they made it look like so much fun here on TV.

On Friday we sit first with Hui Ayi, a beautiful thirty-one-year-old woman from Hebei province. Her hair is long and silky and she wears it tucked behind her ears. My heart soars when she walks in. She speaks good English and smiles warmly when we sit down in the living room. Hui Ayi has just finished three years working for an Indian family who took her to London. I want to hire Hui Ayi on the spot. Then I learn that she can't cook any food except Indian—saag paneer, she says, and the yellow curries her Indian family taught her. I decide we'll eat a lot of Indian food this year. It will be fun, I think—a change.

The key to me seems to be to hire Hui Ayi so I'll be able to go lie down in the bedroom. It's three in the afternoon and jet lag has hit full force. I just want to get this over with. But then Hui Ayi explains that she has a boyfriend who lives in Beijing who works in the far west of the city, a two-and-a-half-hour bus ride away. He will be angry, she warns us, if she's not available to him on Fridays and Saturdays and Sundays. She says she needs to be paid exactly double the amount we paid Xiao Wang. It's more money than I've heard of an ayi receiving. I've always been uncomfortable talking about money, so I don't make any kind of counteroffer. I just hope Hui Ayi will lower her price, but she insists this is the new going rate.

Jennifer Ayi is a tiny sprite of a woman, even thinner than Xiao Wang. She comes an hour after Hui Ayi leaves. My first thought is that Jennifer is so thin she must be sick. But she has perfect fake teeth and a whole lot of energy. She's been recommended by an American woman who, for three years, let Jennifer run her household: paying bills, raising the children, cleaning house, cooking. This is more or less how the ayi world works in China: the ayi is indispensable. The ayi rules the house.

Jennifer Ayi wears a one-piece shorts jumpsuit and a plaid cotton baseball hat. Tufts of her hair shoot out from the sides of the cap. She seems like an instant, though quirky, fit. She was born in Beijing, is fluent in English, and has a great smile, and I'm tired again so I want this to pass quickly. It would be nice if we could get the interview over with so I could take a nap. Except after the first ten minutes with Jennifer, I notice that she has this funny thing she does with her face: each time she finishes a sentence, she opens her eyes extra wide and parts her lips into a kind of exaggerated O—as if she's been startled. Then she looks sideways at some invisible point just to the right of my shoulder. At first I think I'm imagining it. But she does it again. And then again. It's almost as if she's stoned. Tony notices it too. We both have the same concerned eyebrows. We're so ready to hire someone, though. Anyone. It's late in the day and we're on Eastern Standard Time. We want to go to bed. We ask Jennifer if she can start on Tuesday. "Yes," she says and stares off into space with her mouth wide open again.

*Good,* Tony and I say after Jennifer leaves and we make it to the bedroom. We've hired Jennifer. We say we're glad that's settled. We go to sleep, and Aidan wakes up at midnight with jet lag. Then he and I lie in his single bed from midnight until 6:00 a.m. talking about why he can't sleep and how he needs to be touching my face in order for sleep to work. Before, I would have been mad at him for keeping me up all night. Resentful, even. I have more patience now. At least breast cancer has made me calmer. There's no other way to explain it. I lie in bed with Aidan and look back at those years of lost sleep and I can't tell you how foolish I feel for my anger. I used to yell at Thorne for waking me up. I used to beg him to let me sleep. The light is bright on those years. They look like gold from here. At the time I didn't see them for anything close to what they were.

On Saturday morning Jennifer calls and says she's so sorry

but maybe she won't be able to work for us after all. She wishes us luck and Tony and I both admit we're relieved. Xiao Wang comes back in the afternoon with her friend Mao Ayi and announces that working at our house is really easy. She can do all the work in much less time than the six hours we pay for. She confesses she's a terrible cleaner. She hates cleaning. I stare at Xiao Wang and think how odd it is that we've spent so many days together in this apartment, just the two of us—me working at my desk, her talking on her cell phone and searing pork in the kitchen. I never once thought I knew Xiao Wang. But I sensed we had some kind of implicit understanding. The sort between mothers, or rather, between a woman who pays another woman to take care of her kids and the woman who is paid. It's an awkward understanding at best.

Four o'clock in the afternoon: jet-lag witching hour again. It's sleep you can't fend off. I want Xiao Wang and Mao Ayi to leave so I can lie down. We hire Mao Ayi on the spot. It seems like the best way to get them out of our apartment. She doesn't show the slightest interest in Aidan and Thorne, who come and go on Rollerblades in and out of the living room, but I pass this off as first-day jitters. If Mao Ayi and Xiao Wang would just leave, I could lie down and sleep on the couch where they're sitting now. I hand Xiao Wang a wad of hundred-RMB notes to pay her for the work she didn't do in August while we lived in Maine. I also give her a plastic bag filled with Aidan's outgrown sneakers and some shorts and pants for her son. I say good-bye to her and wish her luck. She has a difficult life. Her family is exceedingly poor. I realize I'll never see Xiao Wang again. Both she and Mao Ayi put on their black pumps in the hall and step into the elevator and are gone. It's seven o'clock at night and Tony falls asleep facedown on the couch. I tuck in the children and make it to our bed, where I sleep until 3:00 a.m., when Aidan comes in and settles next to me. He's thirsty, he says. His room's a little scary. He'll do much better if he lies next to me.

On Sunday morning we go to the suburbs and visit our new Danish friends Anna and Lars, who've just returned from summer break in Copenhagen. Their boys, Mads and Gustav, became good friends with Thorne and Aidan at school last spring. Anna is a tall, striking woman—a pharmacist by trade, with snazzy plastic eyeglasses. She is a relief to talk to, so direct sometimes she makes me laugh. On my first date with Anna, we went for a walk in the old hutongs south of Tiananmen and got lost, but she never seemed rattled. We circled the gray maze of stone alleyways, and when we couldn't find the larger road, we got out the map and stared at the street names. An older man approached us and laughed. Then he explained in Chinese that there was a left turn we kept missing back around the bend.

Anna's husband, Lars, works for Nokia. He's a marathon runner who also loves to cook. Today he's bought local grape tomatoes and is making a salsa with Tony in the kitchen. Anna and I sit in the living room sipping wine. Her mother died of colon cancer several years ago. She says, "I've had it with cancer. Completely had it." Later Tony and I have to drive back to our apartment with the boys for one last ayi interview.

Tony greets a small-boned woman wearing a long black dress at the door. She tells us her name is Mao Ayi and takes off her black pumps, then gives me a firm handshake. We walk toward the living room, and Tony quickly explains to me in English that during the Cultural Revolution, families named their children after Chairman Mao to show patriotism. There are now hundreds of thousands of women named Mao in China. It turns out her full name is even more patriotic than the first Mao Ayi's. Tony says the exact translation of this Mao Ayi's name is Mrs. Glorious Army Horse. She wears blue eye shadow and has a quick smile and wants to see the vacuum cleaner and the mop. I take her to the back closet and she nods approvingly at the equipment. I feel I've passed a crucial test.

Mao Ayi #2 lives twenty-five minutes away by bike and knows the small vegetable markets in the hutong behind our house. She meets Aidan when he comes in from skateboarding and follows him into his room to ask him how old he is in Chinese. Mao Ayi #2 does not speak English. But she listens to me when I try to use my Chinese and gently helps me with my verbs. Tony and I hire her because it's getting late again, and I can't keep my eyes open. I walk Mao Ayi #2 to the door and she calls out good-bye to Aidan. "Zaijian, Aidey," she says. How does she know we call him that? She's the ayi for us. *Good,* Tony and I say after we climb into bed. *It's settled.* We're falling asleep, but Tony promises to call Mao Ayi #1 in the morning.

It is now quarter of eight at night. Both boys are asleep. I gave Aidan a pep talk about sleeping when I tucked him in. I told him his brain was ready to make it through the night. That his body now knows he's on Chinese time. He nodded at me. "But what if I need you?" Aidan asked me before he fell asleep. "What if I call out for you?"

"I will always come," I tell him. "I will always come for you. Meiyou wenti: no problem."

# Science Experiment

The first week back in Beijing the skin on my chest turns a dark sunset red and begins to peel. Dr. Godin said this would happen: that it would get redder and tighter after the radiation was finished. Most peeling takes place under my left armpit at the site of the lymph-node scar. Aidan first catches a glimpse while I stand in my underwear and search a drawer for a T-shirt. Today is the first day of school in Beijing all over again. How did Aidan become a kindergartner?

I'm not ready to be here yet—not braced for the dislocation. The boys are unsure too. School in China starts up earlier than in the States, and we pulled the plug on summer in Maine too soon for anyone's liking. There had been a time—a window of two weeks—when I deliberated whether or not to do chemotherapy, and I thought we might stay in Maine and not return to China. I imagined us moving back into our house and envisioned the wooden beds and bookshelves—the scaffolding of our lives there.

During this window, Tony and I drove down to Boston to talk to the doctors again about recurrence rates. We were still deducing how much benefit chemo might give me. "I know where you are," Tony said afterward, when we pulled out of the parking garage. "You're unpacking plates and cereal bowls in Maine. You've moved back into the house and said good-bye to China."

It was a hard moment in our marriage. I wasn't sure if I was ready to close the door on Beijing completely, but if chemo was in store, then the idea of my own bed—of our own home—was not something I could turn away from easily. I didn't know how to answer Tony because what he said was true: I *had* been calculating how many days we'd need to unload the moving truck.

Then he said, "I get it, you know. I completely get it. Of course you'd want to be home. But I'm up all night trying to figure out how we're going to keep our family together. I have to be in China to do my job. We need that job. And I can't live apart from you."

Part of me knew we weren't done with our time in Beijing—that we'd left too abruptly. But home has its own tidal pull, and staying in Maine was hard to resist. In the end we chose not to do chemotherapy—we couldn't find a doctor who said the benefits outweighed the risks.

"Yuck!" Aidan yells at me now in my bedroom. "What's that under your arm? What's that skin doing?" He screams for Thorne to come take a look. This is not the first time I've felt like a science experiment for my children. I'm the different one. I'm the female specimen—the one who has to explain where her pee comes from. "Thorne!" Aidan screams again for his brother. "You've got to come look! You've got to see this!"

Thorne races into the bedroom half-dressed in a white and red Chinese soccer uniform. He's carrying the soccer ball in one hand. "Disgusting!" he yells when he sees me. "That is gross!"

"It's just peeling," I say, trying to act casual while I pull my T-shirt on over my head. "Just peeling skin." I go into the bathroom to wash my face and try not to let my hands shake. They are children. They don't know what they're saying. They follow me and stand close to my waist while I reach for the face towel. It always amazes me how alarmed the boys are by my body since the cancer. Because what is mine is theirs in the world of young boys and my body is in some ways sanctified to them. So how could I let such a thing transpire, and on whose watch? What would they do if I tried to explain the concept of silicone to them? What they want is a return to normal. Not skin falling off in pieces like small leaves.

What we're striving for here is a return to the way things were before—a mommy who's at the bus stop every day. Thorne stares at me in the bathroom mirror. "Mom," he says quietly now. "Mom, you've got to put sunscreen on there." He points at my armpit through my T-shirt—the place where the peeling is the worst. "You just have to."

I look at him and wonder when he became a teenager. "Okay," I say calmly, as if I've never thought of this. As if sunscreen will solve the entire problem. "Good idea. Sunscreen. I'll do it."

Then Aidan says, "Boys are lucky because they can't get breast cancer." Who knew this was on his mind? I nod at him and decide not to quibble with facts. "Mommy," Aidan continues, "did you know that there are one hundred women in the world who get breast cancer who can't fix it?"

"Sort of," I say, hoping to steer this conversation toward a soft landing.

"Yup," Aidan assures me. "One hundred. And that may sound like a lot but it's not really when you think of how many hundreds of people there are in the world."

Then even Tony comes running into the bathroom. What's with him? He's just back from the police station. There's a scary new sign outside the apartment complex that says in English, "All Foreigners must register with police upon arrival. Or the Judicial Organ will affix the responsibility for the criminal acts." Tony rushed our passports over to the station this morning, then realized he needed a different permit to prove the authenticity of our lease, so he came home, then rushed back again.

We're now standing by the shower door, staring at my covered chest, and we're late for the bus. "Can I see the peeling?" Tony asks. Things are getting out of hand. All summer I've tried to keep the whole burned skin situation low-key. We need to get on with the business of going to school. I give Tony a look. More like a plea than a look. He smiles at me— he's realized his slip, and shoos the boys to their rooms for socks and pants.

That's when I hear Aidan ask Tony what his sister, Polly, died from. "She got cancer. Right, Dad?" Aidan says.

How have we come to this sad place on the first day of kindergarten? I almost don't recognize us for the kinds of things we talk about now. "Yes, but it wasn't breast cancer," Tony answers brightly. "Polly didn't die of breast cancer, Aidan." And here's the thing about children and cancer—my children, anyway. They muse on it, then they make their own connections. They don't shy away from the scary stuff.

"She didn't die of breast cancer?" Aidan confirms.

"Nope. She didn't. Not at all."

I go back into the bathroom and the tears come. I think I'm crying for the darker things about cancer that Aidan doesn't understand. I'm swimming in the cancer lake again. Aidan and Thorne are standing on the grassy bank with Tony, peering out over the waves to see if they can spot my head. Today it feels like a long way back to my family.

I peek around the doorway. Aidan leans against the wall in the hallway outside our bedroom wearing his first pair of big-boy jeans. He says, "You can't die of breast cancer. Did you know that, Daddy? You can't." I watch Tony pause, and I'm amazed at the way my husband is able to meet the boys' questions and redirect them. Because how much can you talk about breast cancer at 7:45 on a Monday morning with young boys?

"Aidan," Tony says and picks him up in his arms. "We should go and find some sunscreen in the hall for this face of yours. It's going to be a scorcher on the playground today."

Then I dry my face and walk toward Thorne, who's standing by the front door. I take his shoulders in my hands and squeeze them and say, "I love this boy. How did I get so lucky to have this boy?" and he laughs and swings the door open to the hall. "Let's go, guys," I call out to the three of them then. "Let's go to school."


After they leave, I walk to a café called Jamaica Blue that's opened next door to the French grocery store—right between the high-end antiques dealer and a new dry-cleaning shop. Elizabeth calls me on my cell phone and tells me she's been thinking of me all month. I thank her for the e-mails she sent to Maine. She says she can't believe I came back to Beijing. I remember again how much I admire her bluntness. She's not afraid of asking me how I feel. "I can't believe you came back," she repeats. "I would have never come back."

It's taken me all week to get over the name of this new café: Jamaica Blue. But today I go in and ask for a slice of quiche. Then I sit at one of the shiny black tables with my writing notebook and watch the concrete shops. The New Age singer from Ireland named Enya plays on the sound system. While we were gone this summer a whole section of shops across the street was torn down to widen the road. I can't think this is a good omen for the hutong. I take a bite of quiche and watch a Chinese man do tai chi in the middle of the sidewalk. He pauses and checks his cell phone. A younger man sits on a concrete piling out front with a baby in his arms. He sat in that same spot holding the baby when I went into the market yesterday. The man wears flip-flops and navy trousers and an old black blazer. He's gentle and knows the way the baby likes to be held: hugging the man's thin shoulder with its bare feet in the man's open hand.

My plan is to open my notebook any minute and begin writing, but I can't concentrate. Anxiety has followed me to China. I stare out the window, and the decisions I made about treatment are up for grabs: to chemo or not to chemo? To radiate or not to radiate? To go vegan or veggie or to stay carni? To suppress hormones or let them run wild? And here's another thing, and maybe this is the most important one—there's no one in Beijing except Tony to really talk to about my cancer. None of those new friendships is strong enough. Or maybe I'm selling the women short. Maybe it's me who's not strong enough to reach out to them.

A woman I met at the playground trampoline yesterday comes into Jamaica Blue—a Chinese investment banker who just moved here from Hong Kong with her husband and five-year-old son. She's got a black bag on her shoulder and the big white letters spell C-h-a-n-e-l. She asks me, "What does a person do for fun in Beijing? Is there a Disneyland here?" I'm tempted to tell her I've taken to spending long stretches of time watching the people in the concrete shops.

It's time to go pick the boys up from school with Lao Wu in the van; I promised I would on the first day back. When I get there, Thorne and Aidan are playing soccer with their friends on the field. One mother I know from a cooking class asks me, *Are you okay?* I've decided that when people ask me this and tilt their head, what they're really saying is *Did you beat the cancer? Or have you gone over to the realm of the dying?*

I can do it this way. I don't blame anyone for not mouthing the word out loud. No one on this soccer field knows me well. I nod my head. I say, *Yeah, thanks, I'm okay.* They all go back to watching the game, and I stand there wondering why it feels like a train has just run over me. When I get home, Mao Ayi has left a bowl full of tomato and egg noodle soup on the stove. It's delicious. I watch the boys eat dinner but my mind has gone away. Tony comes home, and I tell the boys, "Mommy's not feeling well tonight." I go lie down in my bed and spend the next three hours wondering what caused my cancer.

It's a dark hole I slip into more and more. And hey—I'm done with the treatment. I should be doing cartwheels. So why am I not floating on air? I think about the Camel Lights I smoked in high school. Did *they* cause my cancer? It's dangerous territory. And what about fruit? What about the apples and bananas I should have eaten more of? And then there are the cruciferous vegetables. What about red bell peppers?

On Saturday morning I decide the answer is to pack up the minivan and head to the Great Wall. We need to get out of the city and hike on top of something bigger than us—a wall that took millions of people thousands of years to build, one that stretches across China four thousand miles. When we arrive in Mutianyu it's still morning, and we rent an old house for the night from an American man and his Chinese wife.

The village is a cluster of a hundred or so squat brick homes built along the mountainside. A dry patchwork of terraced cornfields surrounds the houses, and rows of chestnut trees. The house we rent has a stone roof and elaborate wooden latticework that covers the glass windows. Double doors painted Chinese red lead to a cement courtyard, where we can stand and look up to the watchtowers on the wall. It's good to be out of the city. Aidan and Thorne climb a persimmon tree and holler down. Tony takes pictures of the boys hanging from their knees and then cuts open a persimmon with his jackknife to see the pale meat.

The entrance to the wall is a twenty-minute hike up the mountain from the house. The boys wear Red Sox hats and carry backpacks with water bottles. Tony keeps the black Nikon around his neck. We pass the woman walking her camel. I saw her the last time we were here. The camel looks old and dirty and grumpy. The woman parks him up at the ticket entrance and charges people ten kuai to sit on him.

It's been one year. The wall seems smaller now, less intimidating, like so many things do in China the second time. The sky is blue, and we can see a series of dark green mountain peaks that stretch in either direction for miles. A uniformed guard asks if he can have his picture taken with Thorne because of his straw-colored hair. Aidan asks to buy a Coke from a man selling them in one of the watchtowers. Tony and I say no to Coke on the Great Wall. But we cave in to gum. It's Doublemint, and the boys each buy a pack for three yuan. Down below us are miles and miles of forest. I think I can see the top of our rented house. Thorne tells us to look at the moon. "It's still full," he yells. I take Tony's camera from him and walk toward my children.

"Aidan," I say. "Lean in toward your brother." Then I snap the picture of both boys together looking out over the edge of the world. It's difficult on some days to believe that cancer infiltrated our family planetary system—our sun and moon and stars. But each of us is different for that now. We've survived something together.

Tony takes a sip of water and tells the boys that thousands of Mongols used to attack the wall on horses. "They'd gallop to the edge," he says, "and then the Chinese guards would push them back with swords and bows and arrows." Aidan and Thorne love this part.

"Don't forget cannons, Daddy," Thorne says. "The Chinese army used cannons." At some point the Chinese installed small iron cannons along the sides of the wall. Thorne sits on one that's turned to rust. Then he starts calling out, "Genghis Khan, where are you?!"

What I'm trying to do here on this wall is get some traction. I met a psychologist at a dinner last summer who told me it takes most of her cancer patients five years to come to grips with their diagnosis. I'm beginning to understand what she meant. I pull my water bottle from my backpack. My body now feels like a molecular-cellular mystery to me. Part of some great, biological fuckup. I'm beginning to see that cancer is for life. You beat it back with surgeries and drugs. You beat it with a stick if you have one. You trick it. But even then you're in some kind of dialogue with it. Because you never want cancer to surprise you as badly as it did the first time. We've made it to the other side for now. The four of us are standing on the Great Wall to prove it.

The village of Xiaolumian lies one valley over from Mutianyu, and the next morning we wake up at the rented house and hike over. There's a hand-drawn map that says we're supposed to cut through a field of pear trees, then after the second bend in the road we should start looking for a pig farm. We head down the mountain this time. Thorne leads and Aidan scrambles to stay in second place. Tony follows Aidan and tries to keep him from falling off the side of the steep path. The boys are singing a song about buying Chinese sweets. They like to walk in the woods.

We hike until the path stops in the middle of the orchard. The map says nothing from here. Thorne closes his eyes and points left. Left leads to a small enclosed valley with no way out except to retrace our steps. We shuffle our way down the path to the split again and head right this time. I scan the hills for signs of the pig farm, but I've never seen a pig farm before, so I don't know what to look for.

I've been told that almost every house in a Chinese village has a sow. There are cornfields here, too, and more chestnut trees dotted with green, hairy shells. In one week the farmers will close these paths and carry ladders into the trees to harvest the nuts. We hike the next twenty minutes over the hill and end up in the backyard of someone's falling-down farmhouse. I'm thinking about millions of Chinese pigs and how I never understood the numbers before, when Thorne yells that he can hear animals grunting. The path cuts through a side yard past five pink sows in concrete stalls. They're the most enormous pigs I've ever seen—heavy and unmoving while dozens of piglets root underneath for milk.

There's also a handful of chickens eating seeds at a wooden trough. More chickens. Thorne is scared and runs back to hold my hand. But Aidan charges ahead and the birds squawk at him and flutter in the dirt and I hope he won't reach out and grab one. A Chinese boy opens a red metal door and peeks his head out of the farmhouse. I smile. He smiles back and quickly closes the door. Tony pulls the hand-drawn map out of his pocket. The arrow says to follow the path to the main road, which leads to the village center.

Xiaolumian doesn't have the air of impoverishment of some villages closer to the city—or the smell of being forgotten. Bright red flowers have been planted along the sides of the road. Xiaolumian is the county seat of the local Communist Party. "A model village" is what the sign says in Chinese when we come to the plaza. There's a group of white-haired men gambling with cards at a square concrete table near the exercise yard. It's the blue machinery I've seen in Beijing: one low balance beam, a seesaw for building leg muscles, and a high span of monkey bars. Off to the right is what looks like Communist Party headquarters—a gray brick fortress in the middle of town, with a boulder taller than Thorne out front and the Communist sickle painted on it in red.

We sit down on the bench next to the exercise yard, and an old woman without any teeth comes toward me from an open doorway. She places her hand on my arm and fingers the bright green bracelets I'm wearing—the bracelets I got with Lily in Wiscasset last summer. We bought them and then giant chocolate-chip cookies at the bakery next door. This was after too many hours looking at Andrew and Jamie Wyeth paintings in a refurbished white barn further north. The bracelets are made of recycled rubber, and all the money is said to go to the women in Mali who make them: twenty-five dollars for twenty-five bracelets.

It was the last day of my radiation, and we climbed inside Lily's Subaru to put the bracelets on. Nothing about the summer had seemed funny to me until then: not the mastectomy. Not the odds on how long I'd live. But twenty-five green rubber bracelets is a lot on one arm, and halfway through, Lily and I began to laugh. I don't know what Lily laughed about, but I laughed for how grateful I was for her and for what a relief it was to be with her, miles north of the radiation room.

The old woman is still holding my arm. She points to Thorne and Aidan where they stand on the balance beam counting out loud in Mandarin. "Whoever falls first loses," Thorne says to his brother in Chinese. The woman tallies up the boys: "Yi ge erzi. Liang ge erzi." *One boy. Two boys.* Then she laughs and speaks quickly to Tony, who translates: "She says you should have another child. She says the boys will leave you, but girls will always stay and help." I smile at the woman and hope she'll go on her way, and when she does, Tony and I sit on the wooden bench and hold hands while the boys make it across the monkey bars.

Someone has painted a sign in white on the part of the mountain that sits under the wall. The Chinese characters spell out "Long live Chairman Mao," which Tony reads to me over and over like he can't believe it.

"Oh my God," I say.

"It's fresh paint," Tony whispers.

"An eyesore." I laugh. "Why are you whispering?"

"Because I think this town is a Communist hotbed. We wouldn't want to screw up in this town." The characters stretch across the whole left side of the mountain saddle. Later we learn that the mayor of Xiaolumian ordered the slogan, and that the mayor is, as another man in the village tells us, a Communist zealot. His village technically owns the part of the mountain the slogan's written on. The mayor told the town he only redid a sign that had already been painted up there, and that "Long live Chairman Mao" has sat on the mountainside for forty years while chestnut trees grew up around it. But that was then and this is now, and Mao is dead, and one of the Chinese men we meet back in Mutianyu later calls the new slogan an abomination.

That night, Tony and I and the boys have dinner outside a small wooden farmhouse in Xiaolumian. There are home-made noodles with eggplant sauce and peanuts and green onions on top. There's rice wine and a dish Tony calls shred-ded chicken. Someone has strung white lights in the trees. Aidan announces halfway through the meal that he plans to get a PhD in rocket science, but only to pay the bills while he becomes a rad skateboarder. Thorne laughs and says, "You can't be both a rocket scientist and a skateboarder."

But Tony argues that of course you can be both. "You can always be both." Then we hear thunder and lightning, and Aidan panics—screaming that he's afraid of thunder. I tell him the storm will miss us, and I take him in my lap. But then the rain comes, and we put our chopsticks down and run for the farmhouse. Inside, there's a kang and a circle of wooden chairs. A woman sets down a plate of sliced moon cakes on a table by the door—apricot, coconut, and red bean.

It rains harder now and thunder cracks over our heads. Each time the lightning flashes it feels dangerous and exciting. Tony stands in the open doorway watching the storm. The boys eat the moon cakes while three Chinese musicians come in from the rain and take seats next to us. One man carries an *erhu,* which looks like a long, thin fiddle with two strings. Another man has a *baosheng*—a metal gourd surrounded by thin bamboo pipes. The third man is the singer. He begins a strange-sounding song that rises and falls in a high-pitched, meandering way. Other people have run in here to stay dry, and we watch the musicians. There's a passing moment when I feel lucky. And then the feeling goes.

But I appear to be a healthy mother with two boys in my lap eating red bean moon cake in the mountains of northeast China. What is true and what is not true in cancer and in China is always changing. I learn as I go. The singing ends unexpectedly, and the baosheng player rises to pour a small bit of water down the mouthpiece of the gourd. He shows the boys how it's easier to blow air through the hole when it's wet.

Then the rain slows and Tony runs outside to find a man who'll take us back to Mutianyu by car. We drive slowly because the wet tar is slippery and because hundreds of small toads have climbed onto the road. Aidan sees them in the headlights first—pale, rubbery toads hopping in the rain. He cries, "The toads. Look out for the toads! We will kill them." And it's true. We are driving over toads. But what can we do?

What I remember about toads is that they're amphibians and there's a time in their lives when they breathe both underwater and in the air. Our car keeps moving along, and toads keep hopping in front. It's more than I can stomach—a mass killing of amphibians. So I say Chinese toads are smart enough to hop around our car wheels. Aidan is only five years old. I want to protect him. I don't want any more talk of dying—not of toads or little boys or mommies. I say, "The toads will be okay," and Aidan seems relieved. He nods at me and stares out the window solemnly.

When we get back to the rented house, the boys climb into the narrow beds, and I read them a Chinese folk tale called "The Goddess of the Moon." There's a daughter named Chang E in the story. Her father is the river god, and he sends her to live on the moon as punishment because she says out loud that she wants to live forever. When I come to this part of the fable, I wish I could take the whole thing back and start over with a new story.

Because this is not the Chinese folk tale we need tonight. What we need is a simple story about the good life here on earth. A fable about food, maybe. Something about a harvest and wild animals finding seeds to last through winter. Not a tale about more longing for immortality. Chang E's husband becomes god of the sun so he can be closer to his wife. Then on the fifteenth day of each month, Chang E and her husband are allowed to visit each other on the moon, which is why the moon always shines brighter at mid-harvest. This is when Thorne announces that he, too, would like to live forever. I'm not surprised. I've seen this coming. He lies in bed next to me looking serious. He's seven years old, and why wouldn't he want immortality? Why wouldn't he want to live forever? Or want me to?

All summer he's been suspicious of my cancer. I don't think he fully believes me when I say the surgery didn't hurt because I was asleep. Or that I'm fine now. I say, "Yes. To live forever—wouldn't that be fantastic." This is another one of the techniques I learned from the therapist in Boston. She said sometimes it will be easier for the boys to stop wanting things if I agree with how great their fantasies would be: a new skateboard, a whole pound of penny candy, immortality. The idea is that they'll feel like they almost got their wish—just by my agreeing with it. Thorne listens to me say I think it would be great to live forever. Then he smiles slightly and goes back to staring at the picture of Chang E. In the picture, Chang E is wearing a long red Chinese robe, and she stands alone on the top of the moon.

# No Assembling

We drive back to Beijing on Sunday night, and on Monday morning Mao Ayi arrives to take charge of the kitchen. She gets here at eleven and leaves at six and never stops moving. Like most ayis in China, she wants to be called "Ayi." It's a job that garners respect. Today she tells me in Chinese that she's going to make pork dumplings like she used to at the train station restaurant she worked at. She assures me that the boys will love the dumplings. She says she's heading out to buy new sauces and cooking oils. She doesn't like any of the ones I have. She'll ride her bike and be back in an hour.

Mao Ayi looks fantastic for a woman who's fifty-three. Today she wore a sequined denim bomber jacket and a gray wool beret, then changed into a tunic and leggings after she got here. When she gets back from the store, she shows me the things she's bought: red chili paste and black bean and garlic sauce. Long green onions. Leeks. Many heads of garlic. She takes a bowl from the cupboard and places a large piece of ginger in it, then slides that into the fridge. She talks loud and has a gravelly laugh from the smoking she does. The boys and I stand at the kitchen door listening to her and we're all a little transfixed.

She redefines the word *thrifty* for me. She discovers pieces of old apple and peach I threw in the garbage last night because they were browning and rescues them by slicing and boiling them. Then she offers them to the kids with brown sugar for dessert. She sends a maintenance worker away when she realizes he's going to charge her ten kuai ($1.50) to replace the small lightbulb above the stove. She'll do it herself in the morning, she says, even though neither Tony nor I can pry the plastic casing off to get the old bulb out.

Just before she leaves, Mao Ayi comes into the bedroom to ask where I keep the towels. She sees the charcoal Buddha sketch on my desk and picks it up to study it. Then she asks in Chinese if I like the Buddha. She puts her hands together for prayer and bows her head. I tell her I do like the Buddha. (*"Wo xihuan."*) But she wonders why my drawing of the Buddha is so small. (*"Wei shenme?"*) She has a bigger one, she tells me. She draws the outline of a larger frame in the air. Much bigger. She likes to repeat her words and asks me again why my Buddha is so small. Then she says her son likes to pray to the Buddha. (*"Wo de erzi."*)

After Mao Ayi leaves and the boys go to sleep, Tony and I eat dinner. I tell him I think she's a Buddhist.

"Along with the rest of the nation?" Tony asks me.

"What do you mean?" I say.

"Buddhism has been here for centuries."

"Yeah," I say. "But I thought religion was banned. I didn't think anyone could even talk about religion."

"You can talk about it," Tony explains. "You can go to the temple and light your incense. You just can't congregate. No assembling."

"So you can't belong to a church?"

"Not in the way you and I might belong to a church." Tony takes a bite of the shaved radishes. They are bright red and remind me of candy, but taste like vinegar.

"I don't think I've ever belonged to a church," I say. "And what about Mao?"

"Yeah, Mao sort of shut everything down."

"So it was not okay to have a framed picture of the Buddha in your house during the Cultural Revolution?"

"No," Tony agrees. "You could get persecuted for something like that."

The next morning Mao Ayi arrives at the apartment and finds me in the bedroom at my desk before she's taken off her coat. "Ni hao," I say.

"Ni hao," she answers and hands me a gold-colored calendar with a large painting of the Buddha on it. The writing is in Chinese.

"Xie xie, ni," I say several times. *Thank you.*

"Ni xihuan ma?" she asks me. *Do you like?*

"Dui, dui. Wo hen xihuan." *I like the Buddha very much.* It's so kind of her to give me the calendar that I'm short of words.

She explains how much bigger her Buddha painting at home is. She's still worried about how small the little sketch of Buddha on my desk is. I ask her how her friend's birthday party was last night. She explains that she drank too much. She tilts her head back and pretends to drink from a bottle. She has a headache today, she says. Morning has come too quickly.

At ten o'clock, Rose rings the doorbell. It's the first time I've seen her since we've gotten back from the States. She embraces me in the doorway and then we each laugh. I tell her in English that she looks great. Her hair is longer, and she's changed her glasses. She now has a smaller, sleeker black pair with "Gucci" on the side. I try to tell her in Chinese that I have not studied my Chinese all summer—that I have been *bing le* (sick), except the translation doesn't really work. Because I haven't really been sick. I've felt fine, in fact. I've just had cancer, but I don't know how to say this.

"It's okay," Rose keeps repeating to me as we walk to the couch. "It's okay." Then she asks how I am and tells me she is glad to see me. "Do you have the charm?" she asks me then. "The charm I gave you?"

"I keep it with me always," I say, and she nods, and this is all we mention about my disease.

We sit down and she asks me to repeat after her: Faguo (France), Deguo (Germany), Hanguo (Korea), Taiguo (Thailand), Meiguo (America). We've gone over the country names before, but it's good of her to remind me. She teaches me again how to say "Ni hao. Wo shi Meiguoren." *Hello. I am American.* Then she says her boyfriend can be a little bit of a problem. That he *bu xihuan ribenren.* Which I understand to mean that her boyfriend doesn't like the Japanese.

"Shi ma?" I say. It's the closest thing I know to saying *really* in Chinese.

"Ta yao ribenren hui jia," Rose says, which means her boyfriend wishes all the Japanese would go home. He lives with his parents now, but next month he'll take ownership of a one-room apartment he's bought. "He wants me to move in with him," she says in English.

"Ni yao shenme?" I ask her. *And you want what?*

"I won't move in until we're married. It is the custom here. My parents don't approve of him. And besides," she says, "I'm not sure I ever want to move in. Until we are married, he can leave me and I will have nothing."

"Do you want a wedding?" I ask her in English now. "Do you want to marry him?"

She laughs her nervous laugh. "I think he is preparing for it. He calls me on the cell phone every hour. He always wants to know where I am. What I do."

I stare at her. "I think you are too smart just to teach foreigners like me. Too well organized." I'm convinced Rose could find a diplomatic job if she went back to the States and got a master's degree. "Would you ever consider going to the United States? Meiguo?" I ask. "There are colleges there. Universities I am sure would take you. Maybe a linguistics program? Maybe a master's in international politics?"

Rose watches my lips move. "I am not sure what I want to do. Every day I am thinking on it. No one in China ever talks to me like this. About things I care about." Her eyes well with tears. "Many of my university friends have moved away. And besides," she goes on, "I care about more than just clothes and cell phones like they do."

I don't know why, but I feel an urgency in the room. I want to tell Rose, *This is your moment.* I want to explain that choices will be made for her if she doesn't choose soon for herself: she'll marry the boyfriend and have her one child and never leave. But maybe I'm getting ahead of myself. Maybe Rose doesn't want to leave China. Maybe there are hundreds of thousands of Roses now in China. Millions of young women with college degrees who don't know what to do with them. "Have you thought about teaching young children?" I ask her. She's such a good listener; she'd make a wonderful elementary-school teacher. "In a school?"

"No," she says. "I have never considered any other career than the one I have. I learned English and then I began teaching foreigners. My other friends have office jobs."

"What do your parents say?" I ask. "What do they want you to do?"

"They want me to get a real job in an office. They want me to leave my boyfriend. He did not go to college and they don't think he's good enough for me."

"Have you told your parents that your boyfriend has bought an apartment?"

Rose starts crying now. Silent tears. She says, "I cannot tell them. They don't want to hear about him. My father has had to move to Shanghai. He was running a rubber factory back home but then was forced out. It was political. He was the boss and then he was left with nothing. So he has gone to Shanghai to manage another rubber factory."

"And left your mother alone?"

"Yes," Rose says, and smiles now. She wipes her tears with a small square of tissue from her black purse. "My mother is happy for this. For forty years she has been cooking and cleaning every day for my father—never getting a rest. Now she can take a break." Rose stands up to leave. I walk her to the front door.

"Thank you, Susan," she says then. "Thank you for listening to me. I have many thoughts going around in my mind now. Many ideas. No one else asks me about these ideas. No one here wonders what I am thinking."

# Ecological Farm

Yesterday Thorne asked me, "Which side is your bad side, Mommy?" and then pointed. So I did jumping jacks in front of him, and then we went outside and had sprinting races on the playground. I'm trying to show them that I'm healed. That I'm no different than I was before my surgery. So that's why today I am headed on a school bus with Aidan's entire kindergarten class to what Aidan's teacher is calling an ecological farm.

I'm dreading the day. It's possible that the ecological farm is a sham. Maybe I've already lived in China too long, but just take the term *ecological farm* for a moment. It sounds important, but if you pull it apart, there's nothing left. What farm isn't ecological?

I'm crowded into the last row of the bus with Aidan. His friends sit near us, punching each other in the arms. Other mothers ride the bus and we smile and nod and realize the limitations of our different languages: Cesare's mother from Italy is here; and Villiya's mother from Norway; plus Alexander's mother from Russia; and Josh's mother, Karen, from Taiwan, who reaches across the aisle and offers me a salty dried prune.

The bus stops on a stretch of road inside the farm near a crop of green leafy vegetables. I'm assigned three children for the day: Julian, a five-year-old from Austria; Mona, a six-year-old from Germany and Korea; and Aidan. I know Mona. Last year Mona and Aidan sat together in preschool and drew pictures of people with long, pink triangular bodies. At our apartment we say Mona is Aidan's friend that is a girl. We can't say *girlfriend*. That word is already taboo. Mona's favorite color is pink. Today at the farm she wears a pink dress with pink polka-dot tights and black Mary Janes. Overnight the temperature in Beijing dropped from sixty-five to forty-five degrees. There's a hard wind at the farm and the children are underdressed, Mona most of all, so Aidan and Julian and I hold hands and huddle around her next to the bus.

Our first stop is the bathroom. It's the dirtiest one I've seen in China. I take it as a bad sign. We've been attending Chinese public toilets now for over a year. The boys and I have perfected the squat. At first it was a tricky thing—reteaching a four-year-old and a six-year-old how to go to the bathroom. I remember how I held Aidan by his armpits over the hole in the stinky stall inside the Forbidden City and tried not to fall in. At this farm the toilets are all squatters—brown and crusty with things growing on the sides of the small drain. A row of windows sits above the scummy sinks, and the glass is covered in blackflies. It's as if a few centuries ago, the farm manager decided to walk away from this bathroom and conduct an experiment on what happens to the ecology of toilets and sinks when they're used by troops of schoolchildren, but never cleaned.

Our farm leader is a young Chinese woman who makes me nervous. She herds us toward the fields in one direction and then abruptly turns and herds us back. She carries a small battery-operated megaphone, and each time she changes her mind she yells at us in broken English to turn around. Finally she leads us into a long, narrow greenhouse covered in clear plastic. We walk the edge of a broccoli field and stare at the bushy leaves. The woman yells something at us in Chinese through her megaphone, and a teaching assistant from Aidan's school tries to translate: "She says that this broccoli is organic. No chemicals have been used to grow it."

I look at the garbage on the sides of the fields, and I think of the bathroom we've just visited, and I make a plan not to eat organic broccoli anymore in Beijing. I'm in the middle of a crisis of confidence about China's food chain anyway. The first year I was here, I was able to turn a blind eye. But not now. This month they've discovered melamine in the milk—a synthetic that dairy farmers add to make the milk appear to contain more protein. Six children have died after melamine calcified their kidneys. Hundreds of thousands have been hospitalized.

Yesterday a rumor spread through Beijing that maggots were in the oranges. So the oranges were all thrown out. I've already stopped buying eggs. Melamine showed up there too. Farmers fed it to the chickens as well as the cows. The foreign press thinks the Chinese health officials should check the goats and pigs. The possibilities are endless. The Mayo Clinic says breast cancer survivors should eat pounds of green, leafy vegetables like the broccoli in this field I'm standing in. I try to tell Julian and Aidan and Mona what *organic* means. I say, "Organic vegetables are fed by the sun and the rain and the soil and have no chemicals." But I think my lesson is lost on them. The woman with the megaphone screams at us to head over to carrots in a field nearby. It's ten o'clock in the morning.

We've got a long day ahead, and the children are shivering in the wind. "How do carrots grow?" the voice in the megaphone asks the children in Chinese. The teaching assistant takes the megaphone again and translates. We learn that carrots grow in dirt, and that is the sum total of our ecology lesson.

Then we're left to roam on our own. My little tribe heads over to the birds. Aidan says, "I've been waiting all day to see these guys." The bird pen is a muddy concrete situation that's more disconcerting than the broccoli field. Water and excrement have pooled in places on the cement floor. A collection of sad-looking geese walks gingerly: we count fourteen of them, plus two turkeys, four peacocks, two enormous ostriches, a handful of ducks, and five chickens. The words *avian flu* keep popping into my head. The birds squawk at us until someone from the farm brings over a basket of wilted lettuce for the children to feed to the animals.

We've been told that soon the kids are going to gather chicken eggs inside the filthy pen. *We don't need eggs from those chickens,* I want to say to someone in charge. What we need to do is wash our hands with soap and hot water and go home. Because this is not the farm for us. There are pretend handbags in China, and pretend milk, and now there's a pretend farm. And there's no soap on this pretend farm either. None that I can find. There are two empty swimming pools, though, and a bumper car ride that looks like it's been kidnapped from an amusement park and then left here to rust.

This is a farm that dreamed big and fell short. The teachers decide to cut our losses and leave. There will be no egg gathering, and the farm is too dirty for us to sit down anywhere for a picnic lunch. We get back on the bus and I'm given hand wipes to pass out to the children. "Why aren't we getting to find chicken eggs?" Aidan asks. "I wanted to gather eggs!" He and Julian wait for my answer. Mona isn't paying any attention. She says she's pretending to be a water bug. She climbs down on the floor in her pink tights and hides under the seat, which doesn't seem like such a bad idea.

. . .

Aidan and I get back from the farm, and wait to meet Thorne off the school bus. Then we walk home and I heat up leftover pizza while the boys draw with markers at the dining table. Mao Ayi called in the morning and told Tony she had a fever. Without her here, it's surprisingly quiet in the apartment. It makes me realize how loudly we talk in our new Chinese when she's around.

Tonight is a normal school night in Beijing. Tony is on his way home from the office, and nobody in the apartment is musing about breast cancer. No one is wondering out loud how you get to heaven. I hear Thorne say to Aidan, "It was awful at school last year. I did not know how to draw a star. I suck at drawing." I wince. Drawing is not something I'm good at either, and I'm afraid I've given Thorne bad drawing genes. His drawings, like mine, are one-dimensional and rudimentary: sticklike humans and narrow houses with thin chimneys.

Aidan calls out, "Mom. How do you spell the word *boat*?"

"B-o-a-t," I say and bring the pizza to the table. Aidan shows me his pirate ship and says he's named it *People Who Want to Tear Down the World*. There are small, intricately colored flags on his boat and humans with large-fingered hands. Drawing comes naturally to Aidan.

"Nice work," I say to him, even though I've recently read an online article on parenting that urges parents to be specific in praise of our kids. Apparently, children are getting too used to vague praise, and this is making them complacent.

"So, Aidan." I look at his drawing again and try to back up. "I like the way you drew that anchor in black marker and made it hang down behind the boat."

"It's not an anchor, Mom," he says. "It's a rudder."

*Oh, really?* I want to say. *Oh, please.* Thorne is next to me, busy drawing more stars. His confidence seems restored.

"Here is a perfect star," he says and hands me his paper. "And here."

"What good work," I say tiredly, giving the most vague kind of praise. "What perfect stars." In truth, the stars look rushed and messy and are hard to discern.

The boys finish the pizza and run back to Aidan's room to wrestle. I gather up the drawings on the table. Above his stars Thorne has written, "Thorne does not have a girlfriend." Down at the bottom of the page it reads, "Does Thorne have a girlfriend?"

Later, Aidan rides into the kitchen on his skateboard and finds me finishing the dishes. "Can water feel itself when it's cold?" he asks earnestly.

"No," I say, glad to be able to answer something definitively. "Water does not have feelings."

"What about crabs? Can crabs feel when the water is cold?"

"I think so," I answer and walk out of the kitchen. "I'm going to take a bath."

I get in the tub and close my eyes and try to feel the normalcy of the evening rain down. It is the kind of normal I've been working toward all fall: a state of mind that does not allow for fear. An apartment where my boys talk about the dimensions of stars and no one asks me if I'm going to die. I hear Thorne greet Tony at the front door with a yell.

That's when Aidan jogs into the bathroom, sees me in the tub, flexes his tiny arm muscles, and asks me again if he looks any stronger. "Definitely," I say. "Your biceps are definitely bigger."

I stand and grab a towel, but I am too late. "When are you going to get another nipple?" he asks me. We've gone over this before.

"In June." I'm intentionally vague about the where and the how, and I don't explain that the thing will be fake. Or that later on, someone (a tattoo artist who moonlights at the hospital) will tattoo the areola on me. I have a hard time getting my head around this information, which is why I can't offer it up to Aidan. I almost don't believe it myself.

Aidan looks at me closely. "In June?" he says. "June is summer."

"Yep. When we go back to the States for summer."

"But how," he asks me slowly as he thinks it through, "can you be sure it is going to grow back by then?" It's a reasonable question. But this whole discussion is getting too Freudian for me.

Tony comes into the bathroom and saves me. He asks Aidan to finish a chapter of *Charlie and the Chocolate Factory* with him in bed. Then I'm alone again with my fake left breast in China. We dry off. I put on my brown sweatpants and a white T-shirt and say good-bye to the implant.

Thorne is lying on his bed holding *Farmer Boy,* by Laura Ingalls Wilder. He reports that Almanzo has spent the entire day in the one-room schoolhouse. I turn out the light and lie down on the bed. Then Thorne says he's undecided.

"About what?" I ask.

"I can't decide if I ever want to be ten."

"And why's that?"

"Well, if I am ten, it means I am closer to dying. Except I want for there to be a next week because next week we go skiing in Japan."

"That's true." I take a breath. "And you don't have to worry about dying," I say slowly. "Dying is a grown-up problem."

"I wish I could close my eyes and be back in America."

"Where would you go?"

"To school," he says. "I would go right to school to see my friends. Don't you think everyone in America is just waking up?"

# Starter Buddha

On Sunday I tell Tony we need more help at the apartment—some kind of Chinese talisman to ward off the leftover cancer juju. Because there's too much talk between the boys about my disease. "Too much brooding on life and death, don't you think?" I ask, and he nods. I suspect he would agree with just about anything I said at this point. "I think maybe a Buddha head is what we need." He nods again, and maybe looks slightly resigned to what the coming day will bring, but he does not complain once. No. He seems entirely game. I think he's trying to humor me. Trying to see me through to a healthier place, where I don't have so much anxiety or wake up on Sunday mornings needing to go buy religious artifacts.

It's a mild morning in October, and our kids are at double playdates. How often does it happen that Tony and I are alone together on a weekend in China? Almost never. And since we've made it through the circus that was our summer of cancer treatments, and trips to hospitals to meet different flavors of doctors, it seems natural to me to get ourselves to the biggest flea market in Beijing.

The first one we see is a beautiful Buddha from the shoulders up. He has a large, round head carved from some kind of pale wood, and he's been covered in white plaster of Paris, which smudges on my fingers when I touch his ear. He's really only a head—with long, impossibly wide eyes and full, rosebud lips. There's no body to speak of. I like him. I can tell Tony does too, by the way he's stopped in the crowded aisle to stare.

"That's a pretty cool face," Tony says, and smiles. We're surrounded by Chinese "antiques," the detritus of a city embracing free market enterprise. There are rows of 1940s Mao wristwatches, and red and black feng shui meters. There are brightly embroidered Tibetan booties and slim Communist-era metal cigarette cases. You can buy tea-colored calligraphy scrolls and vintage Cultural Revolution posters of the Long March. You can bargain over wooden moon cake molds and the earliest Chinese radios and glass mirrors with etchings of the imperial family. You can bargain over anything.

Perfectly natural that Tony and I chose to come to this crazy place full of Beijing's castoffs. Because we are in need of some kind of help here. A statue of an animal god or a torn Tibetan prayer flag (we don't particularly care which) to take back to our apartment and help keep watch over the cancer with us. That's what we're doing now—every day without having to say it: keeping watch, making sure it doesn't come back, making certain it doesn't destroy the time we have together. We are knocking on wood. We are eating our fruits and vegetables.

It's a long, mostly invisible vigil—one that I hope lasts until we're old and gray and have forgotten the cancer. But that's why I motion impulsively to a man in a black polyester sports coat who looks like he might own this big Buddha head. I ask him in Chinese to bring it down for us from the high table for a better look. The black sports coat says in English that this Buddha is old. *Very old*. Four thousand Chinese RMB old, to be exact.

And also heavy. Getting him off the table is not easy, but the black sports coat and a friend are able to slowly move the Buddha to a small, metal cart with wheels. Then I kneel in the dirt and rub the top of the Buddha's head with my hand. "Very old," the black sports coat says again. "Very beautiful."

It's important to remember that most things at this market are "very old" at first, and almost double the price they should be. The market's name is Panjiayuan, but locals call it the Ghost Market. Long before free markets were legal in China, vendors would bike here to Panjiayuan and set up in the dark to sell. Then they'd disappear like ghosts when police came around to shut them down.

The black sports coat keeps motioning for Tony and me to sit on two small collapsible stools he's brought out for us, but we stay standing. To sit on the stools would mean we are ready to concede that we want the Buddha. It would mean we are prepared to negotiate a price. But we're not. Because negotiating in China is a hard-learned skill. An art, really. One that Tony and I sorely lack. He and I both know four thousand RMB is too high a starting point for the games to begin. But we have no idea how low a price to counter with.

Soon there are ten people standing in a circle around Tony and me while we stare at the Buddha. It's often this way at the market—I show an interest in something, and the Chinese gather round tightly to see how much the foreigner will pay. "I am not prepared for a crowd," Tony whispers to me, then tries to take a step back. "And we're not sitting down," he says. "I repeat. Do not sit down. Nor are we buying a fake Buddha head for seven hundred U.S. dollars."

"I'm with you." I nudge my way back through the small gathering. "I'll admit I know next to nothing about prices of Buddha heads."

"Big Buddha heads," Tony says and takes my hand. "Too

big. Because this Buddha is large. Very large. We don't need this Buddha. What we need is a starter Buddha. A Buddha we can afford."

"Okay," I say and turn down the aisle toward a cluster of Tibetan teenagers selling wooden altar boxes. Their stalls are right next to those of several Han Chinese women selling identical metal Christmas tree ornaments. Nearby, the Uighurs have cornered the market on fake fur: tiger and leopard and bear. I hope the pelts are fake. They have to be fake; almost everything else in this market is. "Okay," I repeat. "A starter Buddha." Then I take one more look at the Buddha on the metal cart. *Our* Buddha—the one with the obelisk eyes.

I must gaze too longingly, because that's when Tony takes me by the elbow and says, "Number one purchasing rule in China: do not stare at the object you're hoping to buy. Do not show emotional interest of any kind." Then he leads me down an aisle of darkly woven Mongolian carpets and calls over his shoulder to the black sports coat that we're going to look at other Buddhas. Cheaper Buddhas. Tony says in Chinese, "We might be back."

We see many other Buddhas over the course of the next hour. Some are made of hard stone and stand with their legs under them. Some are wooden and kneel in prayer. Several raise their right arm to offer blessings. All of these Buddhas are painted and sanded and burnished to look like antiques, but when I press the teenage vendors, they tell me the statues were bought at a factory in Pingyao and are selling for about three hundred RMB each. In other words, they are starter Buddhas.

The Buddha head I love (because I do love it now) is still sitting on its metal cart in Aisle Five when we walk past again. The black sports coat comes running from a small card game over in Aisle Six when he sees us. He yells out in broken

English: "Think of a price you offer, then make deal. You won't regret. This Buddha, very old Buddha." Then he slips his business card into Tony's hand. We are on our way to the front gates of the market. We seem to have resolve. We appear to be leaving the flea market without buying any kind of religious iconography.

"I'm glad you didn't like the starter Buddhas," Tony says and takes my hand again. "Because I didn't either."

"They just looked fake." I smile and look down at my shoes. What I'm really doing now is longing for our big Buddha head—the one we seem to be walking away from because it's too expensive.

"And who ever heard of paying forty-five hundred RMB for something that was probably made to look old in a Beijing factory yesterday."

I squeeze Tony's hand but don't say anything. It's hard to leave. We'd gotten close enough for me to think we might make a deal, even though leaving without the Buddha is probably a good thing. We would have paid too much, and nobody ever likes to pay too much, especially for things you know are fake. And it's probably not a good idea to link my recovery from cancer to the purchase of an extra-large, super-heavy wooden Buddha head in downtown Beijing.

Though I have to admit, I'd started thinking my cancer might be, well, *easier* to decipher if we had the Buddha's help. Because that's what I need here in China: a little assistance. My cancer, like so many, struck without warning—quickly, in the middle of the proverbial night—and it would be great if someone could give me a hand. If someone could help translate what in God's name just happened to us, and tell me where, by the way, my left breast has gone.

Tony and I walk through the crowds of deal makers and arrive at the high iron gates of the market. There's an ATM, just to the left. It's been installed, I am sure, for people just like Tony and me—people who don't have enough cash in their pockets to secure overpriced Buddha heads, and who are very close to doing the right thing: walking away empty-handed. It is the ATM that calls me back to the Buddha.

"Let's phone the guy and just make an offer," I say to Tony. He stops walking and smiles his biggest smile at me. It's a grin that lets me know he's willing. Because Tony is almost always willing—it's a trait born, he's told me many times, of his very unconditional love for me. But it's also a knowing grin. A grin that makes it clear we're going to get taken to the cleaners on the Buddha. A grin that says he'll play the fool, but only for me. "Can't we call him?" I look back over my shoulder and then raise my eyebrows. "You call him," I smile again. It's a pleading smile. "And I'll get cash."

"Go," he says and gently pushes me toward the ATM. "Go." Then he gets out his cell phone and digs in his jean pocket for the business card.

"The hard part," he says when I'm back from the booth with a huge wad of RMB notes, "is deciding what to counter with." And it's true. We have a problem. The black sports coat started the bidding too high. We have to figure out a way to bring the price way down without sabotaging the deal. The bargaining is probably going to be hard and fast and cutthroat.

"Don't insult him," I whisper while Tony dials the phone. "Don't go too low and blow the whole thing up." I am now officially having an emotional relationship with the Buddha head. I've convinced myself that getting it is going to change things for me. It's going to slow things down, for starters—because life has been moving way too fast since that morning last April when I found the lumps in my breast. Life has been racing and now I'm trying to catch up.

The Buddha head is going to *remind* me of things—which

things, I'm not exactly sure. But good, important things. Buddhist things. Things I've forgotten, because the cancer wiped out a lot of my short-term memory drive. Things I promise I'll learn more about if we can just take the Buddha home. So I am now what is also known as a sucker. Tony puts his finger to his lips to shush me. Then I hear him say, "Ni hao." There's a pause, and I suck my breath in through my teeth. This is the moment of reckoning. Tony will now offer his counter price.

Three Uighur men to our right have just spread two gray animal pelts out on the sidewalk (Chinese fox or wolf?) and people are stepping carefully around them. "Fifteen hundred," Tony says quickly then.

What happens next is that the sports coat agrees to Tony's price far, far too quickly. He agrees without even one moment of hesitation—without one attempt at counter bargaining. So this is how we come to know that our Buddha head is a fake, and that we, as they say in our home country, have been played. If the Buddha head is worth anything close to fifteen hundred Chinese RMB, the sports coat would have bargained much longer and for much more. He would have bargained till the sun set. He would have been relentless.

But once you've verbally agreed to a price in China, it's as good as written in blood. There's no backing out—the only option is to pay up or perhaps (if Tony and I were feeling light of foot) try to make a run for it. But the black sports jacket jogs to the front gates almost before Tony has time to put his cell phone away. The man is panting, and the Buddha head trails right behind him on the metal cart. "What a good price you got," the sports coat says when he gets to us. He's all smiles and encouragement. "What an old Buddha head," he repeats, with wonder in his voice.

I hand him the pile of money and say, "Zaijian." The Buddha may be fake, but he's our fake now, and I'm going to love him. We wheel him to the van, and Lao Wu looks at Tony and then back at me and laughs. Then Lao Wu says in English so he's perfectly understood, "You know it's fake? Fake?" Tony and I don't exactly answer. We all three lift the Buddha up and gently place him in the back of the van—carefully, carefully, because he's fragile and could break. Then we drive to pick up the boys at the friends' apartment complex. Thorne comes out to the driveway from the tall revolving doors, and I walk him to the back of the van.

"We have a new member of our family," I say. "Meet the Buddha."

Thorne stares through the glass and then rolls his eyes and says, "But I don't believe in any gods, Mom," without missing a beat. "Remember, Mom. No gods."

"But the Buddha was a man before he became enlightened," I hear myself argue. "He's different than a god. You'll grow to like him. I know you will. He was once just a normal guy like you. A really good, normal guy." It hits me then, standing outside the van in that hot parking lot, that buying this Buddha head is its own act of faith. It's about choosing to walk on the side of the road where the sun shines. It's about hope. But I don't breathe a word of this to any of them.

I watch Aidan peek in the back window of the van. He grins at the Buddha, and the Buddha smiles back at him. Then Aidan asks, "How old?"

"One hundred years," Tony answers and squeezes my hand. "He's at least one hundred years old."

Aidan pauses and does the math in his head. Then he says, "Guys, that's cool. That makes him the oldest member of our family."

# Beijingren

Rose calls this morning on my cell phone to tell me she's taken a full-time job at the Turkish embassy. Her role is to interview Chinese people who want visas to Istanbul. I haven't seen her since our last lesson two weeks ago when I subjected her to the inquisition on her career plans. I'm afraid I scared her off. Drove her to take a mind-numbingly boring job at a large foreign embassy. But who knows? Maybe the job will be great. It means Rose will have a steady income and health insurance, so I'm glad for her because she sounds happy. "It is good," she says. "I get to write up each report in English. It is very challenging. Many people want to go to Istanbul now. Many Chinese."

When I hang up the phone, I no longer have a Chinese teacher. What this means is that I have time on my hands. And shouldn't I be exercising? Isn't that what the Mayo Clinic's latest memorandum on cancer said: thirty-five minutes of cardio five times a week? What I do in the afternoon is seize the moment—all part of my new post-cancer China strategy. I walk over to the fitness club in Tower Four of Park Avenue and sign up with Tony's personal trainer. His name is Marcus. I've never had a personal trainer before, so I'm just getting used to the sound of this sentence.

In my sneakers I stand one full head taller than Marcus. He cuts his hair so short on top it reminds me of fur. His big pectoral muscles make his whole chest appear fake. I keep wanting to touch it to see if it's a real chest that protrudes over his impossibly small waist. Marcus wears a white Adidas trainer shirt and black nylon pants, and a jade dragon pendant around his neck. He starts me out on the treadmill. There's something about the gym that feels pretend—like we're on a bad Chinese television show. It's a big, open room and hip-hop booms over the sound system. I see at least forty treadmills, thirty elliptical machines, and a large herd of stationary bikes.

The name of the gym is the Ozone Fitness Club. Who would name a health club after a depleting natural resource? But that's the name, plastered on huge signs that hang over the gym. I walk on the treadmill at the Ozone Fitness Club and look down through the picture windows out to the row of cement shops. I work up a sweat while a grandfather walks his baby grandson on the sidewalk. Every now and then the old man stares up at the gym windows. His grandson wears the old-style training pants with a clean split down the backside for easy squatting. A grandmother cooks soup on an open gas burner she's brought into the street. A man and a woman climb from their parked car and open the trunk. The man pulls out a large bag of rice and puts it on his shoulder. The woman lifts up a green watermelon. A rickshaw passes, stacked with apples and oranges and bananas. There is a young boy in the back sitting on the pile of fruit.

The differences between learning Chinese from Rose and training with Marcus are too many to list. But for one thing, Marcus and I talk to each other only in English. I can tell that Marcus likes to practice his vocabulary. The other big difference about sessions with Marcus is that I sweat a lot. He works me hard. I know Tony has spoken to him about my surgery. Marcus understands that my left arm is sore and that I can't fully rotate my shoulder. I asked Tony not to tell Marcus about my cancer. But sometimes it feels like Marcus is staring at me funny, as if Tony told him more than he let on to me.

I've learned that if I don't stretch my left arm, the scar tissue around the implant begins to harden. Marcus stands next to the chest press machine and counts each time I'm able to push the bars out. "Come on," he says at the start, or at least I think that's what he says. His English gets garbled and the words sound more like "Keemon."

I'm able to do ten chest presses while Marcus tells me the Chinese government is very poor. I want to ask him if he realizes that China's gross domestic product is growing faster than that of any other country in the world. Or that the entire globe is fretting about China's trade surplus. I want to tell him that I don't think low cash reserves is the problem of the Communist Party.

He tells me to get a sip of water before we begin the bicep pull. "I am from Beijing," he says. "But I do not look like Beijing people." His teeth are crooked. Several bottom teeth sit piled where they shouldn't be, directly in front of other teeth.

"Why don't you look like Beijing people?" I begin the first repetition. The bicep pull is easier than the chest press.

"Arch your back," he says. "Always arch your back." Then he laughs. "Beijing people are small and sweet. I look like I am from the north."

I know enough to understand that where you're from matters in China. Here are the broadest stereotypes that I've learned from Rose: people from the north of China like to eat noodles. People from the south like to eat rice. Sounds silly, but these are the generalities on which a nation goes forward. Rose always describes people to me by this delineation—

whether they're from the north or the south—as if it explains everything.

"Have stretching," Marcus says now. He leads me to a black bench, where I sit down, and then he pulls on my arms in a way that hurts. I close my eyes. "Good," he says afterward. "Back to the abs." He has a serious face when he is not smiling. I sit down at the abs crunch. "Keemon," Marcus says, and begins counting.

# Yashow Market

Today Mao Ayi would like a photo of the boys. It's the middle of October, and she finds me writing at my desk in the bedroom. "Lai, lai." She motions for me to follow her to the wall in the living room. There are ten black-and-white photographs of the boys that my friend Winky took back in Maine—beautiful pictures that catch Aidan and Thorne jumping off trees and sitting on the steps of my mother's vegetable garden. "Wo yao yi ge," Mao Ayi says and points. "Keyi ma?" She wants one.

To keep? I wonder. Forever? She takes different ones off the wall and considers them: first a shot of the boys when they were three and five down by the float in Phippsburg and then another where they're playing inside our old truck in our Portland driveway. She settles on the photo of Winky's that I love best—the one of the boys arm in arm and shirtless, just after they've finished eating Popsicles on the porch by the ocean. Red juice stains Aidan's chin, and he's laughing so hard his eyes crinkle.

It's the photo Mao Ayi likes most too. She says she wants her son to make a drawing of it. He's an artist, she explains, and makes a writing motion with her hand in the air. I nod to her because I want her to love my boys, and I can tell she's already beginning to. If there's anything I can do to speed up this bonding process, then let's try it.

After dinner, I overhear her telling the boys to hurry up and finish their dumplings because she wants to play badminton. It's become their routine. I get to keep score. It's not that I am unschooled in badminton. It's just that Mao Ayi is better, with a great serve and a spontaneous laugh. The boys need new competition. They've been playing badminton against me for a year. I lie on Aidan's bed and call out: Aidan and Thorne, five. Mao Ayi, ten. It's a good thing Mao Ayi decided to stop working at that train station restaurant. It was a lucky day for us when she walked into our apartment.

The next morning Aidan wakes up and informs me that what he wants more than anything is a jade necklace in the shape of a dragon. He harps on it through breakfast—asking where we can get one. I'm thinking Aidan might need a Chinese talisman like I did. So I make a deal with him. Thorne stays removed from the sordid, back-alley handshakes Aidan and I engage in. But Aidan loves to barter, to push deals almost to the brink (eat three more bites of pork and you'll get a yogurt for dessert) just to see what more he might be able to wring out of them. I promise Aidan we'll go buy the necklace after school. I say I will get him to the goods. But he has to pay for it with money he's been saving in his plastic pig.

Most people in Beijing under the age of thirty-five wear some kind of jade on red thread around their neck. There may not be widespread religion in China yet, but some scholars I've read seem to think consumer culture will give way soon to the "the old ways" of spirituality. Maybe jade necklaces are a kind of harbinger.

They might be for sale in the pedestrian tunnel underneath

the main road out front. It's dark and smelly down there. I walked through yesterday on my way home from Jenny Lou's. Two families were selling bright-colored beads and small brass animal statues. They had the handsome, dark-skinned faces of Chinese ethnic minorities—the scientific description of any-one in China who happens not to be Han. During the time in the eighties that Tony spent hitchhiking in China, he mostly took pictures of the Yi and Naxi tribes and the Tibetans. These were the photos that hung in our living room in Portland. The people in the tunnel were some of the most beautiful on the planet. They wore elaborate head scarves and chunky silver jewelry and slept in the underpass with the goods laid out on cotton blankets. There were jade bracelets down there and brass Buddhas and wooden prayer beads and fake amber. But no pendants in the shape of a dragon.

I sit at my desk and try to rework the ending to my novel. Mostly this means rearranging twenty sentences. But when it's time to go meet the bus, the paragraph isn't there yet. Aidan and Thorne jump off the bus, and I lead them to the van, which Lao Wu has parked outside the main gate. Then we drive down Gongti toward the heart of the shopping dis-trict. Cars are stacked up behind the long traffic lights. I lean back in the passenger's seat and get the claustrophobic China feeling. It's partly a sense of how far I am from home, and also a realization that Beijing is a landlocked capital. This is when Thorne reads my mind and leans forward to say, "Mommy, I feel like the ocean should be just down the street."

"I know," I say and try not to sound too depressed. "It seems that way, doesn't it?"

"But the ocean's not here," Thorne confirms. "The ocean's far, far away."

Yashow is a giant clothing emporium: five floors of Max Mara and Nautilus and Prada and Lands' End and Gucci, all of it fake. Foreigners flock to this place, and so do the locals. Today the parking lot is packed with tour buses. It's always crowded here. Buzzing with sounds of bartering. It always feels like if I'd gotten here an hour earlier, I would have found the deal of a lifetime on silk nightgowns or Burberry rain-coats.

Each of the five floors holds a certain number of dealers. They set up in small stalls—maybe a hundred to a floor— and sell underwear and dress shirts and fabric for sheets and cashmere sweaters and Pashmina. They sell iPods and Xboxes and movie cameras. A sign in the lobby reads: "Jade on Fifth Floor." The boys and I take the escalator, and then hold hands and begin to circle the stalls. We see a table with jade medal-lions and bracelets, but no necklaces. There's another stall full of carved jade animals: frogs and turtles and fish but nothing on string.

Then Thorne takes me by the arm and walks me back to the stall at the end of the third aisle. He isn't interested in jade, but he's willing to help Aidan. The girl selling necklaces here looks seventeen. Most of the girls in the market look even younger. This girl spends all day waiting on customers and playing games on her cell phone. She naps sitting up in the corner on a stool. Aidan stands with his hands on his hips, scanning for dragons. When he finds one, he points to it. "Zhe ge," he says and reaches. "Wo yao zhe ge."

The girl holds the dragon in her hand so it swings back and forth in the air. She tells Aidan in English that the dragon is the symbol of strength in China. "When you put this on, you become more powerful." Aidan listens and nods solemnly. How did we get so lucky? This girl is a sage in the disguise of a Chinese teenager. She smiles at Aidan warmly. She's under-stood him perfectly—his need for a little bit of power. He hands me his wad of wrinkled RMB notes, all his money, and then he turns and waits for the girl to tie the red thread behind his neck.

Afterward, he takes a step back from the table and asks me if he looks more powerful yet. "Yes," I say. "I think you're already bigger." I want him to be bigger. He's too thin—his tall body bends in the wind. I want him to be stronger. I want us all to be stronger.

It's Aidan's money, but I'm still a terrible bargainer. I take the bartering personally, when I am supposed to approach it like a job. Like a math problem. There can't be emotion involved. I start worrying about the girl's home life and if she has a bed to sleep in. So I pay too much. I won't say how much. Let's just say my son now has an expensive jade necklace in the shape of a dragon.

We drive back to the apartment. The traffic is worse, and I try to doze in the front seat. Then we eat dinner and take baths and read stories while Aidan holds on to the pendant around his neck. I don't think he's ever going to take the necklace off. I go into his room to kiss him good night and he's worn it to bed.

# Breast Behavior

In late October my friend Genevieve comes to visit from Maine. We put her in Thorne's room, and Thorne moves to Aidan's top bunk. Genevieve arrives with no map. No list of sites to see. She is a tall, fearless traveler who loves hiking in the woods with her dogs after it snows. I am so excited she's here. A friend living in the apartment with us. A friend to wake up to. Someone willing to sit in her nightgown in my Beijing living room with me after the boys are on the school bus, and overanalyze the possible side effects of smog.

The first thing we do together is drive to a remote stretch of the Great Wall. The plan is for Lao Wu to drop us off at a place three hours east of the city called Jinshanling. We'll hike four hours up and over the watchtowers and then down into Simatai, where he'll pick us up. We leave the city and travel through acres of identical high-rise apartments with no side roads to walk on, just a grid of endless state-planned housing and one enormous Jingkelong market plopped down near the highway exit. This is the New Beijing I keep reading about—the suburban dream that hundreds of thousands of downtown hutong dwellers are being relocated to. Slowly, very slowly, the buildings give way to flat countryside and a series of small, poor-looking villages. There's a purple flower in bloom that reminds me of lupine and a blue Ping-Pong table sitting in the dirt in front of one house.

When we get to the wall, Samsung is running a training session in the parking lot. There must be a hundred Chinese Samsung workers lined up in rows. Each wears a black polo shirt with "Samsung" stitched on it in gray. Some of them carry hand-drawn maps for a scavenger hunt. Genevieve and I stand in the hot sun watching them play tug-of-war with a giant white rope.

Then we take an old gondola to the top of the mountain. I can tell that Genevieve is the perfect China tourist—part mystic, part inquisitor. "Let's see if we can camp out here some night," she says to me before we get off. "I already love it here. I can see why you wanted me to come to China."

I'm glad to have a friend here who understands me and does not say things like, "Why are you still sad when you have two beautiful boys?" Which is what my friend Gretel asked me last week over coffee. I'm still worked up over it. She added, "Why can't you be happy for what you've got?" I could not find a way to explain that cancer doesn't work like that. That cancer is sometimes sad. I wanted to stand in that small café with Gretel and pick the table up and throw it.

The gondola makes me think of ski resorts in the 1970s. It's old and rusty and sways in the Chinese wind. Genevieve says, "I had no idea it would be so beautiful here. You tried to tell me, but I had no way of knowing." There are women on the wall trying to sell things. They carry Cokes and Sprites and Hershey bars in canvas bags. One woman zooms in on me and tries to tell me how old this part of the wall is. She's hoping I'll pay her to be my guide. I say, "Bu yao, xie xie," when she gets out her collections of postcards. "Bu yao." This woman must live in the village down below. I don't begrudge her the chance, but she's not making money off me today. I want her to leave me alone. I'm tired of the way she keeps rubbing my arm with her arm while we walk stride for stride. Tired of telling her *bu yao bu yao. Bu yao.* I am becoming the rude foreigner. "I don't want your help!" I finally say loudly and move away from her.

Genevieve and I walk for hours. It's hard going—the path is steep and narrow and sometimes there are no sides to the wall. To fall looks to me like certain death. The mountains ripple out for miles and there's hardly a house to be seen in the forests. Hardly a road. "You've taken me deep into China, Sus." Genevieve laughs. "Wyo and Graham would love it here." Her two boys wait for her back at home. "They would think about the wizards and sorcerers who live here in caves." We stop and get out our water bottles. Three women selling Evian circle us on the watchtower like crows, trying to sell us more. I remind myself that they're doing their job, and that these women have children of their own they're trying to feed.

We set off again, up steep stairs that take thirty minutes to climb. I use my hands and feet, as if the staircase were a stepladder. That's when Genevieve begins to describe the amazing book she's writing for her two boys—a story about the powers of five sacred stones. Each week she reads a new chapter to her boys, and each week they beg her to write more.

Near the end of the hike, there's a uniformed man at a makeshift gate, which marks the entrance to the Simatai section of the wall. He says we need to buy another ticket to enter. There's a small group of Italians gathered around him, refusing to pay. I think if Genevieve and I just show the man the tickets we bought down below, we'll be able to continue. But the gatekeeper wants twenty more RMB from each of us before he'll let us pass.

I'm out of money. I yell at the guard in Chinese that it isn't fair to charge us more. I try to barge past him, but he blocks my way with his body. "There are no signs telling us we have to buy more tickets," I scream at him in English. "You're just stealing our money." Then I shove him with my shoulder. Damned if I am going to be hijacked on the Great Wall by a teenage guard in an oversized military uniform. And what if Genevieve didn't have forty more RMB in her pocket like she does? What was the guard going to do with us then? I feel the rage well up as Genevieve pulls my arm back. She tells me that she's just going to pay him. "I'm worried he'll get the police involved if we try to make a run for it," she says. "It's okay, Susan. I've got it."

I'm angry now for all the times I haven't had the right ticket in China. Or the correct permit. Or accurate directions. Or the perfect words. I scream more nonsense in Chinglish about how it's not fair that we have to buy more tickets. Genevieve gets out her RMB notes and pays the man off, then leads me away by the hand. I'm crying, and I'm not sure why.

Near the end of the path, we cross over a wooden footbridge that dangles above a river. At the far end there's another gatekeeper who charges us more money to cross his bridge. I've given up. I wait for Genevieve to pay again. I don't say a word about extortion.

This guard has laid sardines near the edge of the bridge to dry in the sun. Maybe he'll eat them for dinner. I think he lives in the small cave I see above the bridge. Maybe I'm out of my mind for yelling about twenty Chinese RMB. What I would like to do is start over and leave as much of my anger as I can behind on this bridge.

The next day, Genevieve and I walk the boys to the bus stop. They're mesmerized by her because she tickles them under their chins and has taken to talking to them in her bad college German. Thorne now calls her his German aunt. Once the boys are on the bus, we flag a taxi to Dashanzi to see the art galleries. We stop for tea at one of the outdoor cafés that sprung up for the Olympics. *Time Out Beijing* has put hip-hop star Kanye West on this month's cover. I flip through the pages while Genevieve looks at postcards she's bought of old Chinese cigarette posters. I learn that Kanye will be in Beijing next month to perform at the Workers Stadium. Then I find a half-page article on breast cancer called "Breast Behavior."

October is Breast Cancer Awareness Month, but I'm not used to these articles. *Time Out* is a magazine that tries to be cutting-edge. It caters to expats and has a contest every season for the best new restaurant in Beijing and a schedule of mixed-drink specials at local bars. "Breast Behavior" sounds like a salacious title for China's Communist Party readers. A title that's trying to sound hip about breast cancer.

Just to the left of the article, the editors have included a photo of a beautiful woman named Mu Yeilang in a sleeveless tunic. The caption says Yeilang is a breast cancer survivor and the founder of Beijing's Pink Ribbon Group. Genevieve is busy watching the Chinese tourists on the street. We've already walked through a show of large-scale color photos of garbage sites near the South China Sea.

"Breast Behavior" says breast cancer diagnoses in China have increased 23 percent in the last ten years. It explains that close to two hundred thousand women in Beijing have been diagnosed. But the tone of the piece is dispassionate, as if it's describing a new weather pattern off Hong Kong. The two authors—a man and a woman—write that the real killer of breast cancer is "ignorance."

Genevieve takes out her pen and begins to write a postcard home to her husband, Tom, and her boys. I don't think ignorance is a good choice of word. There must be a better way to say it. Breast cancer, the authors explain, "is easy to treat," especially if Chinese women would practice early detection methods.

Who are these authors, I want to know. Teenagers? I can barely stay in my seat I'm so mad. It turns out I have not left my anger behind on the Great Wall at Simatai. There is still plenty left for me to sort through on this warm morning back in Beijing. Did the authors think they were writing an article about premature hair loss? "Easy to treat"? I got lucky, my doctors kept telling me. I found mine early. But there's no litmus test to prove that a woman's been cured of breast cancer. There's just the waiting. Waiting and living and living some more.

# Homework

I'm standing on a small patch of cement at the bus stop again, keeping my head down to avoid the bracing November wind. Our friend Ken is there—he's the father of Eric, the sweet boy who first asked Thorne to sit with him on the bus. Ken waves and says, "I don't think I'll ever be Chinese." I nod and try to understand what he means because to me Ken *looks* so Chinese. He says, "I've been talking in Mandarin all day at a work seminar, and my face hurts."

Ken and his wife, Vanessa, are a fast lesson in cultural nuance for me. They sound Chinese and speak it to each other on the phone whenever I overhear them. But Vanessa is Taiwanese, not Chinese, and this is a crucial distinction. Ken moved to Long Island from Taiwan when he was twelve. He's a hard-core Yankee fan who often seems more confused by China's byzantine rules than I do. I keep trying to remember that Ken is watching how things are done here just as closely as I am.

Dawn is also at the bus stop. She's the Chinese Irish woman who warned me to eat organic food last year when I told her I had cancer. She doesn't talk to me much. I'm not sure why, and I try not to think she's avoiding me. "We never see you anymore," I say and stand next to her.

She seems hurried. "It's because we have homework every day. No more playing," she says. Her children are five and three. "Every day it's homework. But Henry likes it," she points at her son. He's small for a five-year-old and wears an eye patch. "But it's hard on me. Because I have to do the homework with him."

For some reason I'm still programmed to initiate small talk with people about subjects I'm not interested in. This is another habit I am trying to break in China. I don't want to talk about homework for five-year-olds. I don't believe in it. I want to go home and make oatmeal for breakfast and click on "Real Clear Politics" to see if Obama's seven-point national lead is holding.

"So much homework," Dawn says. "Sometimes two hours." I think I detect a hint of pride in Dawn's voice. People get pretty worked up about homework in this city. A lot of the moms never think their kids have enough of it.

"What school do the kids go to again? I forget," I ask Dawn.

"Yew Chung," she says.

"Oh, right," I say. "I've heard it's a hard school. It's Chinese, right?"

I'm thinking about how Thorne and Aidan's school has clear homework parameters: fifteen minutes a night for first graders, twenty minutes for second graders.

"Yew Chung is an international school," Dawn says to Ken and me. "They have testing."

There's another woman at the bus stop—a Chinese American mother from New York City. I wave to her as she pushes her one-year-old home in the stroller. She told me last week that she pulled her six-year-old daughter, Autumn, from the American school in the suburbs. "They weren't doing enough learning," she explained. "They were playing too much."

Flora is also at the bus stop. She asks me what Aidan does after school. Her English is tricky to decipher, but I know she understands everything I say. "Aidan plays with me after school," I say. "Eight hours is a long day for a five-year-old. He's tired."

"What time," she asks, "do the boys go to bed?"

"Early," I say. I know she'll think I'm crazy, because every Chinese mother I've had this conversation with thinks my kids go to bed scandalously early. "Seven thirty," I add, and wait for her surprise. The Chinese kids here tend to go to bed late, and they're often asleep on the bus in the afternoons when it pulls in. It's hard to wake up from a deep sleep on a school bus at four in the afternoon. It tends to involve a lot of crying.

"Seven thirty?" Flora says and opens her eyes up wide. "Very, very early."

"And the girls?" I ask. "What time?" As far as I can remember, Maggie is nine and Samantha is six.

"Nine thirty or ten," Flora says.

It is my turn for surprise. "Aren't they tired?" I ask. "What time do they get up?"

"I have to wake them," Flora explains. "Every morning I have to shake them."

"What," I wonder out loud, "do they do all night until nine thirty?"

"They eat and do homework and then they pray."

Flora is more religious than I thought. They have family prayer after dinner? Flora goes on, "On the weekends there is no homework. The girls pray all day. Pray and pray and eat. Sometimes I tell Maggie she is like a pig. All she does is pray and sleep."

Surely the girls are not that religious? Then I realize this must be a case of the missing *l* in Mandarin. *Play and sleep.* That's what Flora is trying to say. The girls are playing every night before bed. Finally another family that is having a little fun.

On Sunday, Sabrina and Nick come for lunch. I haven't seen Sabrina since we took the kids horseback riding. Nick is still living in Hong Kong, commuting back to Beijing every weekend. We sit down to a buffet of cold cuts. Today was the first time sliced turkey was for sale at April Gourmet. I bought some, plus mozzarella cheese and an avocado and a baguette. It cost a small fortune to put on this Americanized version of a French lunch in Beijing. The avocado was five U.S. dollars. The cheese cost seven. I pass the tomatoes to Tony, who smiles. The tomatoes are from China and were cheap.

Nick says Sabrina is overscheduling their children. It's part of an ongoing feud. "It's the Chinese way," he says. "She works the kids into the ground."

She tries to explain why her daughter, Rachel, has three hours of homework each day. What I know is that Sabrina has her kids in piano class at 9:00 a.m. on Saturdays. Then she has them in math tutoring, English-speaking class, or Chinese writing class every day after school. "She's behind," Sabrina announces, then reaches for the cheese. "Rachel is way behind in Chinese." This is difficult for foreigners like me to understand. How could Rachel be behind in Chinese? She speaks Mandarin fluently.

But the Chinese parents need more than that. Understandably, they need their kids to write the thousands of Chinese characters fluently. I try not to take sides at lunch. I say, "Our kids are just too tired for tutoring after school."

Sabrina asks Tony if the boys use the playground outside every day. "Most days," he says and looks at me and smiles.

"While the Korean and Chinese children are doing their homework." She laughs.

I'm getting paranoid. Because then I say, "Well, they don't play *every* day. Thorne does his homework before bedtime, and sometimes we have special drawing time together."

Sabrina asks if I have any after-school tutors for math and reading. It's never occurred to me. "Not just now," I say and try to change the subject.

"It must not be that interesting for your kids here," Sabrina adds. I don't understand what she means. "They already speak English, and that's what everyone is trying to learn here."

"Oh no," I say. "Aidan and Thorne are learning Chinese. They like learning Chinese. It is very interesting to live here. Every day they write and speak Chinese."

"Really?" She asks. "How is that?"

"It's Tony," I explain. "He speaks and writes Mandarin. He makes it fun for the kids."

"No Chinese tutor?" Sabrina asks.

"No tutor."

# Foreign Intelligence

Today is November 4 in China. I go to a treadmill at the gym and turn on CNN on the small attached TV. We're twelve hours ahead of the States, so the voting hasn't begun yet in Maine. Obama has opened up a twelve-point national lead, but some state races have gotten closer in the last day. Marcus stands next to the TV screen and watches with me while I run. He says, "Obama will win today. It is historic. A black man winning your presidency. He is very dark."

"I know. I know." I can't think of what else to say. I'm too nervous. When I've done my ten-minute warmup, Marcus motions toward the abs curl. I hate this machine more than the others. I've never had strong abdominal muscles and I do not see the need to start trying now. Marcus begins to ask me a question about Obama, but he can't come up with the words he wants in English. He gets out his cell phone and looks up the Chinese. Then he reads the translation to himself. "Susan," he says, "are you in Obama's *political party*?"

"Yes," I say. "I am."

"Oh." Marcus smiles. He's impressed in some way I cannot understand. Then I realize we're having one of our misunderstandings.

"But Marcus," I say, "our political parties in the United

States are not like yours. Anybody can be in a political party. You get to choose which one you want and then you're in."

"Really?" He seems shocked.

"There are no interviews. No questions. You just register to vote and check the box that says Democrat or Republican or Independent or Green."

"And then they decide whether or not to let you in?"

"No. You're just in." This will take a while to register for him.

"And you can change parties?" he asks me.

"Anytime. You can always change."

"Wow." He laughs. "Crazy."

"But most people don't change because they like their party. And they like the ideas behind their party. Tomorrow"—I'm panting now—"I'll go to a big party at a hotel to watch the election results on TV."

"We do not have anything like that," Marcus says matter-of-factly. "You get to see if the man you like, Obama, will win. We don't get to do that here."


The next morning Tony and I drive to a fancy Chinese hotel ballroom where the American Chamber of Commerce has set up televisions that take up an entire three-story wall. It is 8:00 p.m. in the States and the polls are just closing. Tony and I and hundreds of other Americans eat fried rice and drink Sprite and cheer each state win. Elizabeth is here wearing a T-shirt that reads "Obama Mama."

She's been one of the lead Obama organizers in Beijing—staging voter registration cocktail parties for American expats and hosting house parties to listen to Obama's China advisors on speakerphone. Many members of the Chinese media are here, taking notes on American democracy at work.

The reporters surround Elizabeth, and she finds herself giving interviews all morning. I'm impressed by how calm she sounds. How reasonable. When CNN finally calls the election for Obama, everyone around me cries.

That night Tony and I go to a birthday party in the suburbs at Anna and Lars's house. Anna is turning forty. She wears a long black Chinese tunic and asks everyone to serve themselves tapas in the kitchen. I think I have forgotten how to make small talk. I haven't been out to a party like this since my surgery. I feel the social jitters—as if no one here will ever understand me, even if they did speak my language.

At first, everyone is chatting in Danish, including the German couple we know from the boys' school.

"Congratulations on your new president," a friend of Lars's named Hendrick finally says to me in English.

Anna's friend Mileana adds, "I am so relieved Obama has won."

"Me too." I smile back and can't think of what else to say. I did very little personally to elect Barack Obama—I gave some money and wrote a few e-mails. But I can't take responsibility for Obama's election, much as I would like to. In the kitchen I thank Lars for the fact that he and his friends are speaking English to Tony and me, and he looks at me as if I'm crazy. "In Denmark we are a country of five million people, Susan," he says. "We have no choice but to speak English."

It's a small party, maybe twenty people—men in sports shirts and women in short skirts or wide-legged pants. Lars keeps bringing out bottles of expensive European beer—Duvel and Chimay—and pouring them in Tony's glass. Tony is uneasy. He whispers, "When you're the only Americans at a party, you don't want to be the first ones drinking the fancy beer."

Anna lights three candles in the center of the table, and

during dessert her friend Pia, who's sitting next to me, takes one and pours liquid wax in her mouth. Everyone screams, but her husband just smiles from across the table. "She did this the night I met her, when we lived in Dubai," he explains. Then we all wait for Pia to do the thing she does inside her mouth with the burning wax. It takes a long time. Everyone keeps talking in English, but I feel like I'm missing some key piece of information—some clue to the larger conversation. What is she doing with that wax in her mouth? Is this a Danish party trick? I can't tell if the divide I feel is cultural, or if it's something larger, to do with the boundary lines of cancer.

Then Pia's husband says matter-of-factly, "She can also crush ice and spit it out into cups for cocktails." It turns out that tonight Pia has poured too much wax and scorched the top of her tongue. The wax has to cool inside her mouth before she can make it into a cube. A man who says he operates a Danish shipping container company asks me, "Did you cry during Obama's speech?"

"Yes, I did." I smile, grateful for his curiosity. "It has been a good week to be American again," I say then.

"Exactly right," the man agrees. "After your long spate of imperialism."

The next day I buy two air mattresses and carry them up to the apartment in their cardboard boxes. Lily will land in Beijing this afternoon with her husband and their two girls. I sit on our living room floor and plug the air pump into the wall. It sounds like a loud industrial sander. The mattresses are shiny blue, and when they come to life, they remind me of inflatable rafts. I try to imagine Lily materializing in the apartment and lying on one.

At five o'clock the boys and Tony and I stand at attention in the crowded international terminal. It's always loud in here—buzzing with the emotion of so many different kinds of separation and longing. Hundreds of people hungry for reunion push to see who will be next out of the customs doors. And there's Lily. She's pushing a luggage cart and has a huge smile on her face. Her long blond hair hangs down. Then there's Tyler with his steady gait. He gives a small wave. Their younger daughter, Eloise, is next, wearing her sweet, sheepish grin, and then Calla, my tall goddaughter—who takes everything in.

We hug, and I grab Lily's hands with both of mine. We count the bags and then walk to the parking garage and climb into the van for the drive back to the city: Thorne and Aidan with the girls in the way back, Tyler and Lily and me in the middle seat. I have to keep looking at her to make sure she's real. I'm so hopeful for her visit. Tony sits in the passenger seat and asks Lao Wu if we can go to Ritan Gongyuan, an ancient city park not far from our apartment. Our friends are so tired from the long flight, but we need to keep them awake long enough for them to eat dinner.

Lao Wu stops outside the red gates to the park, and we walk along the path to an old altar where they used to sacrifice animals. It's circled by a high stone wall. There are gnarled willow trees and square stone tables where loud groups of men huddle smoking over card games. Tyler has a smile on his face. "China," he says loudly for emphasis. "I've been imagining this country for a long time." Then I remember that ever since I've known him, he's been fascinated by Chinese culture—hoping to get over here, turning over an idea he has for a novel set in the Chinese countryside.

Lily stares at the altar. "How long ago did they stop murdering animals up there?" She laughs. "And are those blood-stains fresh?" The children climb up on the platform and jump down to the ground. We stop at a restaurant inside the park and Tony orders the house specialty: platters of roast duck. They come with stacks of thin pancakes and saucers of sweet plum sauce. Thorne and Aidan show the girls how to wrap the duck up in the pancake and eat it like a small burrito. I smile at everyone. I'm so glad they're here. But I'm also detached. I think it's the fear that sometimes does this to me. I sit with my chopsticks in my hand, eating from a small bowl of rice, taking in each word everyone says, and then it's with me again—electric blue and zinging. A kind of palpable dread. I can taste it. Not dread of cancer exactly, or the R word, *recurrence,* but of something else. As if I've done everything I could to keep the bad news at bay and I'm sitting in this restaurant eating duck to prove I'm okay, but I'm afraid the bad news is coming for me anyway. It's nothing I can say. Not to Lily or Tyler. At least not on this, their first night in China. And I reach for my Tsingtao and lean back in my chair and try to listen to my friends talking.

In the morning we drive to the Confucius Temple in the hutong south of Houhai Lake. The grounds are empty, and the place feels like a beautiful urban secret. Ancient stone carvings dot the courtyard. Lily and Tyler and Tony and I stand in the temple where Confucius prayed daily. "It's so quiet in here," Lily says. "So calm."

When we leave through the front gate, a short older man approaches us selling calligraphy scrolls. Tony says no thank you in Mandarin, but the man persists. He wears thick, Coke-bottle glasses. We gather around to look at his brushwork, and he invites us back to his house to see more.

"Lai, lai." *Come.* He motions for us to follow him.

We have to hustle to keep up. "Guys," I say, corralling the four kids in the alleyway. "We'll need to be careful with our bodies in this man's apartment." His home sits inside a courtyard house in the hutong that's been partitioned over the years into closet-sized rooms with enough space for a bed, a desk, and a chair. The children sit on his bed and the rest of us stand in the crowded doorway. There's a white toothbrush and a bar of soap on the sill next to the door. The man walks in small circles trying to find the rest of his scrolls. He can't stop grinning. There's no heat, and he wears dark quilted pants and a Mao jacket buttoned to the top to stay warm. He explains to Tony that he was a teacher for thirty years at the middle school down the lane. He's missing most of his teeth.

I remember what Hans said at dinner back in April—that Tony was inside the conversation here and the rest of us non–Chinese speakers were out. I'm glad again to be married to someone who's in. Because this old man makes beautiful drawings, and what a gift it is to be asked inside his home. Tony buys two of the small scrolls for eight dollars apiece. One reads, "To long health and longevity." The other characters spell out "double happiness."

The next day we head to the Temple of Heaven to see the sundial where the harvest prayers were made to the gods. And then on to the Summer Palace. And then the Great Wall. Each day is epic like this—we go to a different piece of history in the city, and the sky stays remarkably blue. "I thought China would be so different. So much more Communist and bland," Lily says on the fifth day while she and I eat dumplings alone at Din Tai Fung. Tony and Tyler have taken the kids to a swimming pool near the apartment. "It's so complicated here," she says. "So much history staring you in the face. We should have planned to stay longer. My God—the girls like it here so much, we should live here!"

For one moment I allow myself to imagine Lily staying in China. But then just as quickly I let the image go. I take a sip of tea and feel the separation again. I realize I've hoped

Lily's visit would spring something loose for me—something to shift the cancer balance. We sit in the crowded dumpling house and I see, perhaps for the first time, that no one is going to do that for me. Not Lily. Not Tony. I smile and say, "It's confusing to feel alone while you're here. It's like I'm waiting for something to happen. Waiting for you to do one simple thing that is going to close the door on the cancer." I can say anything to her, and this in itself should be freeing. She puts down her chopsticks and listens. "It's weird," I go on. "I don't get it."

"I do," she says then. "You're still figuring out the disease. I can watch your mind sometimes trying to solve it—"

"I feel like I've stalled out. Like I've taken some kind of long detour and I want you to understand, but I don't have words for this separation. It's like I've gotten lost."

She nods her head. Then she says, "But you haven't. You're right here. And Tony and Thorne and Aidan are still at your side."

On Saturday morning she and I drive in the van with Lao Wu to see an acupuncturist. Britta has recommended Dr. Heng, and Lily comes because she wants to check things out. She's never had acupuncture before. Neither have I. She says she'll finish reading a novel she's brought in her bag while I'm treated. When we step into the tiny lobby, I'm led to a room by a male assistant and asked to lie down in my sweater and jeans on a narrow cot. Dr. Heng enters then. He has a handsome face with alert eyes. He holds my wrist and listens to my pulse. Then he says, "Your body has had some great event."

I nod at him and wonder how he's discerned this from my heartbeat. I haven't told him about my medical history. He goes on, "We have to tell your body it's over now. We have to tell your body it's okay to let go."

Then he begins to chant a song that repeats the word *bod-*

*hisattva* over and over while he slips needles into my calves and my feet. The needles hurt more than I thought they would. I lie there and listen to the singing and feel the needles humming and wonder if things can get any weirder in China and if I am going to cry, and if this is the final thing I've been waiting for. The healing moment. When he's done, I tell him I've been lifting weights with Marcus at the gym. "You are thin," Dr. Heng warns. "You're not meant to be lifting weights. Only swimming, yoga, and belly dancing." I nod my head and try to imagine me and the belly dancing, but I can't. Maybe this is not my moment and I should go.

Back in the lobby, Lily sits in a chair against the right wall, sobbing. "What's wrong?" I ask, alarmed. "Are you okay?"

Then she laughs and says, "This book is so damn good. But God it's sad. It's about a father who doesn't have a job or money for his wife and kids. He thinks he's failing them. And he is. But then he stops himself. Just before he crashes out, he pulls it together." I stare at her in wonder at her ability to be so moved by a book in this crowded little lobby. I would like some of that emotion. Can she just give me a scoop, please? I would like to feel connected like that again to a book. To a person. To an idea. "The ending is so real," she says, and tears fill her eyes again. "It's so believable."

We walk outside and climb into the van to go home. Everyone is back from the swimming pool, and the kids play hide-and-seek in the bedrooms. Tony and Tyler sit with their feet up on the table, drinking green tea and planning the dumpling house they're going to open back in the States. They've been designing this restaurant for years. Tyler says, "We'd have to get Lily and Susan to work the front of the house for us. Seat people and pour the drinks."

"Yeah, because we'd be out back working our asses off in the kitchen." Tony nods and takes a sip of tea.

"That is a lot of dumplings to make every day," I add and sit half on Tony's lap.

"And just for the record," Lily says, looking over at me, "Susan and I will *not* be going into the hostess business."

"But don't forget naps," I say, standing up now. "Aren't you people tired? See you in an hour." Then I walk down the hall to my bedroom. We're planning to go to a noodle-making class tonight with the kids. It's at a cooking school Thorne's art teacher opened in the hutong. I lie down on my bed and the phone rings. It's Sebastian, our lawyer friend.

"Can you and Tony make it to a dinner tonight?" he asks. "There is an American senator in town."

"Senator?" I say. I knew he had friends in high places.

"We'll meet you guys at Li Qun Duck at six."

"We have our own friends visiting," I say. "Writers. We can't come." But a senator. The idea intrigues me.

"Bring them," Sebastian says. "We'd love to meet your friends."

I hang up and go stand in the hall and make an announcement. "Drop the noodle plans," I yell. "I'm calling the baby-sitter. We'll make noodles tomorrow. Tonight we're meeting a U.S. senator at a duck house in the hutong behind Tianan-men."

"We're what?" Lily calls out from where she's lying with Tyler on the air mattresses in the living room. She says the mattresses are surprisingly comfortable to sleep on, and I can't tell if she's lying.

"High-ranking," I call to her, like it's perfectly normal. "And her husband. We're meeting them in two hours. Are you game?"

"How can I not be?" she yells. "It's too good to pass up."

Then I go lie back down on my bed. Sometimes it seems that since we left the United States, the country has actually begun to get smaller. So small, in fact, that on a Friday night we find ourselves headed to a quarter of the city known as Dongcheng with one of the senior members of the Foreign Intelligence Committee.

"What do you wear to meet a senator?" Tyler calls out before we leave. "I only brought jeans to China."

"I'll find you a shirt, man," I can hear Tony say from the kitchen, where he's making the kids popcorn. "Maybe a sweater. If we can find you a sweater you'll be fine."

Chloé arrives at five thirty and we head out in the van. Part of me wishes I could explain to Lao Wu who it is we're going to see. I want him to know one of our leaders is here. That our two governments are talking. But I can't think of a way to tell him that won't sound self-important.

"We have to be careful about what we say," Lily decides then. "How much can we talk about? How much Obama?"

"I'm going to ask her a lot about foreign policy," Tyler jokes.

Tony grins back. "Yes. Let's talk about two of our specialties, dumpling houses and the Monroe Doctrine."

"Oh God," Lily groans. She's giggling now. "I know this will be hard for you to hear, Tyler, but the senator has not come to China to get badgered with your questions about the Iraq war. We have to be tactful."

"And exactly what is our line of questioning?" I ask and begin laughing too.

"She's come to meet with U.S. ambassadors and Chinese leaders, Tyler, not two writers from Yarmouth," Lily adds. "Please, please promise that you'll ask her politely."

"Yes, please." I repeat one more time. "Because Sebastian and Margaret are our friends. Sebastian hasn't asked us out so we can embarrass him."

"I'm on it," Tyler says. "No worries. There are just a few

things I'd like to say about the sale of our aircraft carriers to Taiwan."

"Oh no," I say.

"No worriers," he repeats and smiles.

Lao Wu drops us off at the mouth of a long, unlit hutong alley. It's windy and cold, and when we open the door to Li Qun it's dark inside and crowded. When my eyes adjust I see dozens of dead ducks hanging by their necks on the back wall. The hallway is lined with pictures of Bill Clinton and Madeleine Albright and Henry Kissinger. Plus a collage of lesser-known American senators, who've all eaten here. I spy Sebastian, talking to a waiter. There's a petite woman standing next to him. I reach them and say, "Hello there."

The senator leans toward me so we do an awkward half air kiss, half embrace. I feel like I know her, and what a peculiar thing—this false intimacy she must try to convey. Or maybe it's not false. Maybe this is how she acts all the time—warm and grounded. The round table we're led to is in a small, tired private dining room. The walls are smudged with dirt, and the tablecloth is greasy. I get up and find the toilet out beyond the open kitchen where the ducks get roasted in a wood-oven fire. This bathroom is so much worse than most of the public ones I've been to in Beijing that I wonder what Sebastian is thinking bringing politicians here.

Back at the table, the senator says quietly that she's just gotten back from a fact-finding mission in Kabul. I stare and try to nod like I'm right there with her, weighing the military options we have against the Taliban, but really I'm studying her hair. How does she keep it in place? I can't pretend to have any expertise about the Taliban. I'm wondering when Tyler is going to jump in.

Sebastian is to my right. "I love this place," he says to me. "Best duck in the city. I always come here." I nod and try to clean my chopsticks off with the hem of my sweater. Why is it so dirty in here? We're all a little nervous, I can tell. Then I look over at Tony. He's smiling his widest grin—the kind I think are called shit-eating grins. He's staring right at the senator, and I hear him ask her how her flight to China was. But her husband is the conversation master. He's charming and funny and soon Lily is talking to him about the plot of her second novel.

The night really goes to Tyler, who in the end, after several beers, begins firing the questions he warned us he would. "Are you here to gauge China's military buildup? And do you see the troops as an inherently bad thing?" Tyler persists. "Because I think too many people fear China when they should just learn more about it. Maybe ignorance breeds fear."

I try not to stare too hard at the senator when she answers. I feel none of the remove I've had earlier this week. This conversation is too surreal to stay removed from. The senator. Right here.

Tyler's voice begins to rise. He's getting emotional and heated, which means he's breaking one of the cardinal rules of talking policy with a senator at a dark and dirty duck dive in an old corner of Beijing. "Why should we fear them? What have they done to us that would make us distrustful?"

I look over at Lily, and her eyes are wide. She's staring at her husband. I try to change the subject by saying to anyone who will listen, "Did you know that Lily's second novel was featured in *People* magazine?"

"Oh really?" Margaret says. "That's fantastic."

Lily looks over like she wants to strangle me. She hates this kind of attention. I can tell she's really mad. But I was only trying to take the attention off Tyler. That's when Tony asks the waiter for the duck carcasses to be brought to the kitchen and chopped up with a cleaver. "There is a Chinese tradition," he says to everyone, "of sautéing the bones with garlic."

In minutes the waiter hurries back with a heaping mess of cooked duck bones. The plate makes its way around the table and we all try a bite, cracking the small bones in our teeth.

"This is disgusting," I say. What a gross idea—cutting up the carcasses and eating them. Everyone is laughing now. In this China moment, everyone is inside the conversation. I laugh so hard that my eyes fill with tears. I haven't thought about cancer for hours.

When Saturday comes again, Lao Wu drives us back to the airport. Up until the moment we say our final good-bye, I keep thinking Lily will find some way for them all to stay. They've liked China so much—every single one of them. Our lives will be quiet in the apartment when they're gone. Lily hugs me and thanks me again. "It's been one of those life-changing trips," she says. "And I hadn't expected it. Wasn't looking for it. I want to come back to this place. To this amazing country." Then she adds one more thing, and it's what I hold on to after she's left.

"Sus." She speaks slowly, standing on the curb of the departures terminal. "I've been waiting to say this all week." She pauses. "I know you're struggling. Reaching. I know you are thinking. All the time still thinking about your disease, and I'm not sure you can think your way out of cancer." I nod at her; I know she's saying something important. Something I can't quite find my way to yet. "Maybe this is the time to let go and just be," she goes on. "Maybe it's not the time to think."

# The United Nations
# of Second Graders

It's difficult to figure out how to celebrate birthdays in this city. But on November 27, we reinvent the birthday party wheel. Thorne is turning eight. We can't have all the kids to the apartment. They won't fit. Who could have predicted that by this time Thorne would have so many friends in China? Or that he would join the swim team and the soccer team and love them both? Or that he would tell me that he thinks he'd like to stay in China until he's a teenager?

Who could have known we'd have this good kind of birthday problem on our hands? So what we do this year is invite seventeen boys and one girl (Molly) to a soccer game at the school gym. It's the United Nations of second graders: Korea, Taiwan, China, England, Bahrain, Cameroon, the United States, Denmark, and Germany are all represented. They play for an hour while Tony runs around with a whistle on his neck, refereeing.

When the games are over, we break for lunch at the Noodle Loft around the corner from the school. Tony blows the referee's whistle to stop and start the herd of eight-year-olds as they run down the block. Eighteen kids at the Noodle Loft gets a little crazy. I pass out a box of metal magic rings I picked up at a kiosk under the pedestrian tunnel last Friday. The kids play with the rings for about two minutes and then begin drinking Sprite through their noses.

Thorne's friend Simon's birthday is also today. Simon's father e-mailed me four days ago and asked if Simon could have his birthday party with us. I told him to join in, but maybe we could keep the numbers below twenty. Because what on earth do you do in Beijing with twenty eight-year-olds?

Tony had asked Simon's parents to take care of the food at the restaurant while we manned the soccer at the gym. "Just order the noodles," I'd said to them as they left. "The kids love noodles."

That was our plan—simple bowls of noodles. It is a *noodle* place, after all. But then platters of duck start arriving. "It is Simon's favorite," his mother explains to me. It's a tricky thing to serve whole roasted duck to hungry eight-year-old boys. There's a lot of food preparation. Too much. Tony and I get busy cutting and distributing meat and thin pancakes and plum sauce. Thorne's friend Ali comes to the party late and with no warning and brings Rashid, his eleven-year-old brother. I smile at Rashid and recall that he is the boy who taught Aidan and Thorne the concept of "getting sexy." What a gift. I tell Rashid to grab a seat too (he has a sweet face) and this bothers Thorne. He says, "The party is getting out of control and Rashid is too old to be here." This is how I learn it's a delicate thing to introduce a fifth grader into a second-grade scene.

We seem to recover, and I make a point of never looking Thorne in the eye again during the party, because each time I do, he makes a mad face at me. There are things about mothering I'll never understand. It's the weight of it—the subterranean pull between my children and me. How can I set Thorne off with a look, when I'm the one who dreamed this party up and invited all these kids? I stay away on my own side of the room, handing out duck to Gustav and Mads and Eric. Each time I sneak a look over at Thorne he's playing with Jiho and making farting sounds with his hand under his armpit while he eats his noodles.

After the party Lao Wu announces that he's taking the boys to a live animal market to buy Thorne a turtle. How can we say no to such a nice offer? He parks the van in a crowded street not far from his own apartment. Then he tells us he keeps two turtles at home, and that we will like having turtles. They'll grow, he says in Mandarin and spreads his hands in the air. *Hen Da*.

Lao Wu takes Thorne's and Aidan's hands, crosses the street, and strides into the crowded outdoor shopping center. Luckily, this is not the live reptile market I've heard about where snakes are for sale. It's a market for tropical fish in glass tanks and hundreds upon hundreds of turtles. How will Thorne ever choose one? Tony and I walk behind the boys, and we circle the entire market twice. I'm not sure what we're looking for—what characteristics mark a good turtle from the rest of the lot. This place is dark and smelly and surreal—dozens of men and women sit inside their tiny stalls arguing the case for their own turtles. *How can you tell the difference?* I want to ask. The turtles all seem to be stoically swimming for their lives in giant, scummy glass aquariums.

Lao Wu looks like he's enjoying himself. He doesn't let go of the boys' hands, but he pauses from time to time in front of certain stalls and gazes up at the stacked tanks. Then he points out a yellow-bellied turtle and then later one tinged a darker shade of green. Thorne finally decides on a member of a hardy-looking troupe of lime-colored, palm-sized turtles. Lao Wu asks the vendor how much. Then he scoffs at the price and the two men go back and forth negotiating the sale of this one little guy who's running in air now, suspended by his shell in Thorne's small hand. Of course Aidan wants a turtle now too, and how can we deny him when the price is much better if you buy more?

When we get home, the turtles will not give any of us the time of day. I can tell that they don't like us. Every time we put them down on the wooden floor they scramble frantically. And who wouldn't? It dawns on me that we've got new responsibilities here. We've got two turtles we have to keep alive until we exit China, when hopefully we can give them away. Thorne puts them in their glass bowl near the sink in the living room and they instantly shrink into their shells.

"Tony," I call out. "I'm glad we finally found a use for the wet bar!" Then Thorne sprinkles brown food pellets into the water and watches each turtle poke his neck out of his shell to swallow. Aidan wants a naming ceremony, and I tell him to think on it and we'll vote at dinner. Then Tony comes out of the bedroom smiling. He likes the turtles. We have pets now in China. Some of us are feeling more and more at home here.

# VI

# Hall of
# Preserving
# Harmony

交泰殿

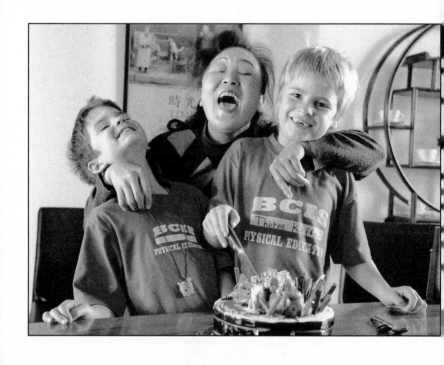

Mao Ayi and Thorne and Aidan in the dining room in the
Park Avenue apartment in Bejing

# Homing Pigeon

In early December my mother comes to Beijing for three weeks, and every day is like a small celebration. Every day is like a holiday. We don't get much family all this way around the hemisphere. "She's here!" both boys say when they get off the bus and spy her standing there. *She's here!* I say to myself. She's tired, too, but what better time could there be to play a full round of Monopoly than after you've just flown thirteen hours up and over the North Pole? We go back to the apartment. She will sleep in Thorne's room—he'll sleep on Aidan's top bunk again.

Thorne lays the board down on the rug in the den. He asks Nona to dole out the money. She doesn't remember that each player gets six of the twenty-dollar bills, not five, until Thorne reminds her. Aidan wants to be the thimble and grabs it first. Thorne chooses the dog. I will be the iron, and my mother is the car.

Things move quickly. I land on Baltic Avenue—it's cheap and I buy it immediately. Aidan seems to have caught on to my strategy. He gets ahold of two railroads within the first ten minutes: Reading and Pennsylvania. Thorne runs into trouble. He lands on the 10 Percent Luxury Tax and has to pay two hundred dollars to the kitty. The boys are getting used to having a grandmother again. They take turns in her lap. She gives them all her attention and they bask. The apartment feels like more fun now that my mother is here. She's come all this way for us, and maybe she'll take some of this mothering load from me. Because I can carry it, but with a little help from her I might be able to put the worst of the cancer behind me.

There is this sadness that's still following me. I don't know where it came from. I wasn't expecting it, and it won't let me go. What I know is that people and things that used to make me happy, sometimes now make me weep. It's as if I'm still trying to understand the cancer. I don't know yet that my sadness is right on schedule. I don't know yet that there even is a schedule.

It's Aidan's turn when I hear a small thud outside the big double window. I don't look up from the board. Aidan rolls double fives and tries to decide whether to buy California Avenue. Thorne thinks he should—it's a great property, he says. My mother mentions casually that a bird has just banged into the window.

"Oh," I say and hand Aidan two hundred dollars for passing Go. "A bird?"

"Yes." My mother stands up. It takes her a moment longer than I remember to straighten out her long body. She is a tall woman—almost six feet—and wears her gray hair cut in a line along her jaw. She has smooth, young-looking skin. "A bird most definitely flew into your window."

The boys and I rise slowly now too, and then the four of us climb over the couch on our knees to have a look. We lean into the window and crane our necks to see the concrete shelf down below. That's where the homing pigeon stands. He's downy white with a long, black-tipped tail and wing feathers that look soft and clean. The only thing that moves on him is his oddly curved head. The head bobs and turns entirely around so that his body faces forward but his head is staring straight at us. It's a bit creepy. The bird's head is covered in white feathers too, though they're shorter than his wing feathers and give the effect of an old, balding man.

"A BIRD!" Aidan yells nervously. "THERE IS A BIRD!"

"He's so big!" Thorne screams. "How did he get so big?"

My mother laughs. "It's beautiful," I decide. "And enormous." Like a city pigeon from downtown Boston, where I lived for many years, but on some kind of growth hormones. It's also stunned because of the crash. Perhaps more problematic is that it's all alone. The little I know about Chinese homing pigeons is that the flock is where it's at. The birds are not supposed to go solo when they're out with their posse. The flock flies as one.

Aidan takes another long look at the big, white bird and then he unhinges. There is no way to explain why Aidan cries, really, except that the sight of the bird with its round bobbing head and avuncular beady eyes scares him. "Wow," I have time to say before Aidan's screams drown out my voice. "Wow. What a pigeon."

I will admit there is something scary about the bird—maybe it's the size. Maybe it's how unannounced its visit is. We've been preparing all week for my mother. Adrenaline is high. We've already got the transatlantic visitor we've been hoping for. And now this strange bird? Aidan's shrieking is the kind a small child makes when he's lost control. "Aidan," I say in a singsong voice and take him in my arms. "Aidan. Aidan. Aidan. That bird is not going to hurt you. The bird is not going to come in this house."

Thorne laughs then, but it's a nervous laugh, as if he's not sure if he should cry along with his brother. My mother and I exchange a look. It's one we've practiced over years. It's such a relief to have someone in the apartment in China to exchange the look with, I almost don't care about Aidan's crying. The pigeon is eerie and peaceful-looking at the same time, if that's possible. Perhaps we've been so starved for wildlife in China that we're in a state of collective shock over the pigeon. Where has this bird come from? And why us? Why now?

The pigeon looks like it's been sent to our apartment with a purpose—a little old man who needs to gather his thoughts and then he'll begin to explain. I hold Aidan in my lap on the couch and rock him until he quiets. I'm about to put him down on the rug. Thorne is back at Monopoly. It's his turn and he rolls a three and a five, which makes eight.

That's when Mao Ayi walks into the den with her hands covered in dumpling flour. She's making traditional Chinese jiaozi for my mother—one kind filled with glass noodles and tofu and egg, and then another with pork and green onion. It's no small thing for Mao Ayi that my mother is here. For days Mao Ayi has been asking what she should cook on my mami's first night. That's what she calls my mother—my "mami." And Mao Ayi has still not gotten over how tall, how incredibly tall, my mother is. In Mao Ayi's eyes, it's like some matriarchal giant has arrived in our midst. Mao Ayi is not sure what to do with my mother's height. Height equals power in China. The Chinese put a great deal of importance on how tall people are—it can dictate whom they marry and whether or not people think they're smart enough to go on in school. My mother has claimed all the power in the apartment simply by walking in tall.

Mao Ayi stands in the doorway and asks in Chinese what the yelling is about. "Yi ge niao," I say in Mandarin and point to the window. "Wo men kan kan yi ge niao." *We all take a look at a bird.* Mao Ayi leans over the back of the couch, and when she makes out the shape of the pigeon down below, her eyes light up. It's a look I haven't seen before from her.

Things happen fast after that. There's no warning. Mao Ayi sees the bird, and then she reaches for the handle on the window and goes after the kill. "Hao chi!" she yells with a huge smile. *Good food.* Before I can stop her, she's opened the window and is waving her right arm at the pigeon, trying to catch him by the tail.

Aidan begins screaming again. "Bu yao!" he cries loudly. *Don't want this.* It's a primal scream. Mao Ayi is trying to trap dinner with her bare hands and Aidan does not even bother with the English. "BU YAO!" he yells again. For some reason he's decided this pigeon means harm. What fascinates me, besides Aidan's fear, and besides the fact that Mao Ayi would like to eat the bird if she caught it—let the blood run in the sink and pluck its white feathers—is that my five-year-old is screaming in Chinese without translating first. "Bu yao! Bu yao!" he says again. *Don't want. Don't want.*

I need to take action. I can't let Mao Ayi get this bird in her hands. I reach and pull her back from the window. Then I turn the handle closed, lock the casing, and say in English, "All done. It's all over."

Thorne is crying now; I think only because the whole scene has been exhausting to watch. My mother takes him in her lap, and I bend down again for Aidan, who's lying in a heap on the rug. Who knew a pampered bird (because that's what it is—it's no visitor from the wild; this bird has come straight from someone's plush pigeon den) could arrive and set the boys off like this?

Grabbing pigeons off window ledges and boiling them for dinner isn't something we've experienced. The boys and I have never seen a bird beheaded. Someday I think this will be important. I'll want Thorne and Aidan to understand where their meat comes from and to imagine a food chain leading to their dinner plates. But I don't think this December night in

Beijing is the right time for a live kill. I smile at my mother again and raise my eyebrows. It's easier to be calm around these children when I have a witness. Because they are sort of driving me crazy now and if my mother was not here, I might yell at them. So often what I think I've needed in mothering is just a witness—someone to make a small acknowledgment. Someone to say, *A bird just flew into your window.*

I smile at Mao Ayi and point to Aidan and explain in Chinese that Aidan is too tired to look at the pigeon anymore. *Hen lei.* She says that the bird would make good pigeon soup if I would allow her to catch it. She makes a tut-tut sound between her teeth, like I'm blowing a great chance here. Like she can't believe I'm going to be so thickheaded as to let this bird go. She kneels on the couch again, watching the bird, and doesn't take her eyes off the window while she talks.

I clarify things. At least I think I do, but there are always moments in China that get lost in translation. How could they not? I say we don't want pigeon soup for dinner. *Bu yao.* I say we aren't hungry for that kind of dinner. I remind her of our plan to eat dumplings. Then I motion to her that I'm going to close the curtains.

"Goodness," my mother says. "My goodness." She smiles at Thorne, who is back in her lap, and then she says to Aidan, "Aidey, I thought you would love the bird. I thought you loved animals."

I worry that my children have changed and that in the haze of cancerland I've missed the signs. Maybe living in this polluted city for too long has given them pathologies about simple things like pigeons that land on our window ledge in the afternoon. I smile at my mom anyway and I say, "It's all fine. It's fine. Fine. Fine."

Except it's not, really. It hasn't been since the day I found those little breast lumps. In fact, there are many things I still don't understand. Like why the pigeon flew into *our* window, and why we happened to be playing Monopoly at the moment the bird arrived. We could have been anywhere else in the house and would have never known the pigeon was down there, gathering itself for flight.

I'm sure my cancer felt like this to my mother when she heard the bad news—a surprise that she had nowhere to place. Tony told her on the phone the night after the surgery here in China. I could not talk to her. I was too sad. There was no context for the cancer. No family history. No bad health. It's as if cancer should fit into some larger story, but it doesn't. It won't. And this is also part of the sadness. Where did the cancer come from and why did it come for me?

This is what my mother did when I got cancer: she waited for us to fly back to the States for the next surgery, and when we arrived she gave my boys bedrooms in her house in the town on the river. She fed them pancakes and cereal every morning. She baked them cakes. She turned her dining room into an art center—with pens and crayons and markers and glue sticks with purple glitter—and she did paintings with them on her big wooden table. She bought Wiffle balls and bats, and she set up a baseball diamond with my father, and together they played hours of Wiffle ball each day. My parents drove the boys to another town where they could learn how to play tennis. They needed things to do. We'd pulled them from school. I was often at the doctor's office. My mother and father drove them for grilled cheeses and onion rings at the Fat Boy drive-in in Brunswick, then let them have ice cream before bed.

Mao Ayi nods at me while I pull the curtains closed. I sneak a look down at the ledge: the bird has begun to pace, which I take as a good sign. We need a healthy bird. A pigeon that is able to fly away. We can't have this bird die on our watch.

We've had enough talk of dying lately. It will be too much. But then Mao Ayi loses control and makes one more lunge for the window. "NO!" screams Aidan, this time in English. "NO BIRDS IN THE HOUSE!"

"Okay!" I yell. "Okay now!" I lean over again and I grab Mao Ayi around her little waist and pull her back toward me on the couch. She laughs but still doesn't look like she's given up. She's lived in a Beijing hutong all her life. Made it through Chairman Mao and the Cultural Revolution. To my mind, the only reason anyone her age in Beijing is still alive is because they are immensely resourceful. They know how to survive. Which means, first off, that they know how to find food. Who can blame her for recognizing a good homing pigeon when she sees one?

She finally stands and heads to the door. Then I pull the curtains closed again and say to everyone in English, "This pigeon needs some rest now. This pigeon needs some peace and quiet." *And let's hope, for God's sake,* I say to myself, *that this pigeon is gone before morning.*

But it's December in Beijing: cold and windy and the bird does not go anywhere. All evening we check, my mother and I, while the boys take a bath and put on pajamas and get in their beds for stories. Each time I look down, the bird is in the same spot. Then things get worse: he stops moving, which I take as a bad sign. This bird is going to freeze to death if he stands still like that all night out there on the ledge. Tony comes home from work, and I show him the pigeon. Then he and I and my mother begin a vigil. We seem to know without saying it that the bird has to live. It has to. But what else can we do but look at it? The window ledge is several feet down, and since Mao Ayi lunged for him, the pigeon has moved to the side, out of reach. Tony finally puts some raw hamburger meat out on the ledge, and a small plate of sunflower seeds.

While we're sleeping, a light snow falls over Beijing, and when we wake up, the city is covered in white. Before the boys are out of bed, I run to the den and pull the curtain back quickly. The pigeon is still down there, and yes! He's alive! Except now he's got some bird friends who've come to visit. Two of them—pigeons just as big as he is, with plump white bodies and long black tails. Where have they come from? And how did they know where to find their friend?

I close the curtains and give each boy a bagel for breakfast and pour them apple juice. With them it's like the bird never existed. I take their cue. We do not talk pigeon. What we talk about is how Nona is going to visit each of their classrooms today at school. Then Tony takes the boys down to the bus, and my mother and I finally pull the curtains wide. The pigeon (our pigeon) sits on the window shelf and listens while his friends balance across the way on the telephone wire. I am not making this up. His two friends call over in some kind of pigeon speak. I believe they tell him there's a way back to the flock, that it won't be that hard. That he can get over this—he just has to follow them.

All year the boys and I have watched flocks fly in formation above the hutong, and we never understood how prized the birds were. How coddled. The pigeons always take a tight path, up through the tops of the willow trees and then down between the nearby high-rises doing loop-de-loops and wing-dixies. We've seen white pigeons and speckled gray pigeons and pigeons the shade of charcoal. The plumpest ones look more like mourning doves. The smallest ones look like American sparrows.

I didn't know these birds have been around since the Ming dynasty, when they were used to deliver messages. I didn't know there are sanctioned pigeon races now: from Shanghai to Beijing, with big prize money. There are over three million homing pigeons in China. A whole pigeon cottage industry. A national pastime. My mother sits in the den on the couch taking pictures, documenting the conversation. "Friends," she says and takes a photograph. "This bird has got friends. They are trying to rescue him." Then we both walk into the kitchen for more coffee. This is beyond anything we imagined.

When we go back to the window, the sill is empty. Poof. The pigeon has gone. And right away, I miss him. Until then, I'd been unsettled. Strange visitor. Unannounced guest from birdland. I didn't know what the bird wanted with us. Now we'll never see him again, and I'm filled with strange longing. I know Mao Ayi will think the bird was a missed opportunity—another example of my willingness to waste good food. But that pigeon was not hers for the taking.

Time moves ahead. Are the boys more easily startled now by the unexpected? Has cancer done this to them? Has China? Or maybe this is just the way they've always been around strange animals and I've forgotten. Cancer can do this—erase some of the time before the cancer, so I'm never sure what's the same and what's been changed. What's been imprinted.

# Israel

The day after my mother leaves China is sad, more so because I have an appointment at the international hospital where I became a professional breast cancer patient. The lobby is an innocuous-seeming place. There are long white couches covered in fake leather and blond wood coffee tables and English-language magazines. But this is the place where the lumps turned out not to be cysts, and the surprise of that fact does not wear off. I am here for my quarterly exam.

One of the Chinese nurses calls my name, and I follow her into the tiny windowless room where they take vitals. The girl wears a set of sky blue scrubs and a blue cardigan. Her hair is pulled back in a dark ponytail. She looks maybe twenty years old. She tells me to take off my coat, then asks why I'm here.

I knew she would do that. But I don't want to answer. I can get snippy about this. I have no desire to tell this stranger the history of my cancer. I will never see this nurse again, and I've been through this conversation enough in Beijing to realize that the nurse wants to know because she wants to know, not because she's going to be able to help me.

I look at her and then for some reason, I give up the fight and say, "Breast exam. I'm here for a breast exam."

"Are you having pain in your breast?" she asks slowly in halting English.

"No," I say. Which is sort of not a lie. I will not talk about cancer with this woman. I will not let her induce me into some kind of truth session.

Then the girl mentions that I'm wearing a beautiful ring. "Where did you get it?" she asks.

"It's from Israel," I answer, impatient. I do not want to talk about my ring. I want to see the doctor and find out about the new densities in my right breast that I'm afraid I felt in the bathtub. "The ring was made in Israel," I repeat. In fact, I met the Israeli jeweler who made my ring the day I bought it. She was visiting Portland and brought her things to a funky craft shop my good friend Jenepher owns there.

"Are you from Israel?" the nurse asks me now. Her line of questioning is the main reason I don't like to talk about much of anything with the Chinese nurses. I know I'm defensive. But sometimes it seems that once you get onto a subject—any subject—it's hard to get the nurses to stop.

"No," I say. I really don't want to be having this conversation.

"Where is Israel?" she asks and finishes taking my blood pressure. "One twenty over ninety," she reads and writes down the numbers.

"It's in the Middle East," I explain. I glance at her but her face is blank. I realize she has no idea what I'm talking about. I spread my hands out on the table. "Pretend my hands are the Middle East," I say. "You know, Iran is here, Iraq is right next to it, and then Egypt and Israel."

The nurse stares at my fingers unknowingly. Then she says, "I think Israel must be a very small country for me not to have heard of it."

I lean back and take a breath. It's alarming to me that the

nurse in charge of vital signs at Beijing's top international hospital does not know that Israel is a country. What do they talk about in social studies in Chinese schools? Do they ever look at maps? Globes? I am grumpy. I don't like this place. This is the hospital that employs the Chinese surgeon who told me I was a worrier.

So does this nurse know anything about the persecution of Jews? Or about the millions of Palestinians living in refugee camps? Has she ever heard of the Holocaust? I'm alarmed. This nurse has got to be one of the more educated women in China. My mind races with the other things citizens of the world's largest population might not know: important things like the gas showers at Auschwitz or what it means to have a First Amendment, or the names of countries like Rwanda and Sudan. Or how it could be that the world's biggest Communist country is home to the highest number of millionaires and the best-selling Mercedes-Benz dealership in the world. I am overwhelmed at the efficacy of the Chinese totalitarian state.

But I'm getting carried away. I am losing my edge. I shouldn't have come to the hospital. I should have stayed home. "What is your height?" the nurse asks me.

"I only know it in inches," I say flatly. I want to blame her now for something. Anything. I want to hold her culpable. I want to tell her that my height will have absolutely nothing to do with whether or not I get cancer again and won't she just drop it? Won't she leave me be? Doesn't she understand that the thing I most want to know about my cancer is if it will ever come back.

I often try to tell myself I've done my job. I had the surgeries. I did everything the doctors asked me to do, and then I asked for more. And she has no idea what it's like to wonder if it's going to return. To wonder is something hallucinatory—a black, unsettled fear—something to stow deep in the trunk and send to the bottom of the sea.

She reads my chart and says nicely, "You are one hundred eighty centimeters. You are very tall. In China we are short people. If you were Chinese, you would be a basketball player or a model." That's when I return to my senses. This petite nurse is not my adversary. Even I can see that. And how unfair I'm being. She sticks a thermometer in my ear and announces with a smile that I do not have a temperature.

I go back to the lobby to wait for the doctor and run smack into my Israeli neighbor. I haven't seen her in weeks, and isn't this unusual—we were just talking about her homeland. She has two sons. Sometimes she sits on a stone bench near our apartment building and smokes cigarettes while she waits for the school bus. Today she appears to have cold sores on her lips and chin. We smile at each other. I begin to consider explaining to her what Israel does and doesn't mean to at least one Chinese nurse I know in this hospital, but what I really want to do is sit down and gather my wits.

I'm done with the vital signs. Done trying to explain where Israel is. I'm nervous. The Israeli woman is here for cold sores and I am here for breast cancer and never the two shall meet. I feel like I'm on a distant sister planet to the planet other people in the waiting room live on. But who knows who might be dying in this small room? Or who is about to discover they have a disease? I can't presume to know anyone else's difficulties—a realization so basic, but the one piece of learning that has deepened my experience more than the rest.

The nurse calls my name, and I follow her into a larger examining room. Dr. M. gets to work right away—kneading my breasts like pizza dough and running her fingers over them in circles. There have been changes in the right breast. Densities. I was right. It is the beginning, the doctor says, of fibrocystic disorder. What does this mean to me in Beijing at two o'clock on a Thursday? Not very much. It means we will watch the right breast—the real one—just a little more closely.

Next a nurse comes in and begins to set up for my six-month Zometa infusion. This is the drug that helps my bones now that I suppress my ovaries and there's no estrogen to feed them. The nurse seems stern at first. She tells me to get comfortable in her broken English, but when I lie back on the bed, she grabs my arm and tells me, "Not yet, not yet. I still have a lot of things to get ready." She has a pretty face with freckles, and short-cropped hair that makes her look like a boy. She has to hook the IV bag on the pole and prepare the needle. Finally, she motions for me to lie down. Then she examines my veins for a long spell. When she finds one she likes on the side of my wrist, she slides the needle in expertly. "You will be here for half an hour," she answers, and sets the IV drip to a speed she likes.

Then she looks down at me and adds out of nowhere in her monotone English, "You are a brave woman. You are strong. I see your happiness on the outside. But I know inside you hurt." I nod and stare at her through my tears, and then she leaves.

# Top Gun

"Marcus," I say, trying to get my mind off the weights he has me lifting. It's a Saturday afternoon in February. "How did you come to work at the Ozone Fitness Club?"

"I went to college to become an electrical engineer," he says in English. "My father was one before me. But while I was in school, I began bodybuilding. No one was doing this in China then. The gyms were terrible. There were only three in Beijing. Bad equipment. None of these machines." He points to the treadmills lined up along the windows. "I worked on my biceps, triceps, and chest. A new gym opened in a complex called Soho. I went there and I looked so good, the owner asked if I wanted a job."

"You left your old job?" I ask. "Wow."

He nods. "It was very big. I did not know what I was doing, exactly. I made mistakes. No one was training in China. You have to understand. The only thing people began to do was to try to look good—to make their muscles bigger. Slowly we learned about proper technique. We learned this from the Americans then. They were very good. Now not so much, but back then, the Americans were serious and the training was good."

"How did you leave your old job?" I open my water bottle and drink.

"It was an easy job. All the factory jobs are easy like that here. Maybe you have four or five men, but very little work. You make tea. You sit and talk. You do not do much work. It is easy but boring."

"Isn't that changing now?" I've never asked him so many questions before.

"Yes, China is moving faster. The jobs are changing. The young people," he says, "are used to the speed."

"But the old people," I ask. "What is going to happen to them?"

"They are all retired. They sit and play cards, and I think they're bored. They don't have religion like we do."

"Religion?"

"Yes, you know that when Mao Zedong came to power, he said religion was not good. Do you know who Mao Zedong is?"

"I know," I say.

"He stopped all religion." Marcus bends to adjust my seat lower on the back press. I have to do thirty of these presses before the next break. "Nobody could be religious. So my parents, they have no religion. But me, I am religious."

"You are?" I'm surprised. "What religion are you?" I push the weights back again with my feet so that I am lying almost prostrate on the machine.

"I am a Buddhist," Marcus says with a smile. He seems proud. "I am a Buddhist, and now we can have religion in our lives again here."

I stand up and take a sip of water. "Are you still writing your stories?" he asks, except I can't understand the words at first. I stare at his mouth and he makes a motion like writing with a pen in the air.

"I am." But I don't want to talk about my writing. I'm at the gym to work up a sweat. To forget about writing and the state of my mind and the status of my cellular, molecular bodily makeup.

"Every day?" he asks then. "Every day you write?"

"Almost every day," I say.

"Now we go work on abs," he decides out loud. "Abs and lower back. Follow me." He sets out across the gym toward the Nautilus machines, walking on the balls of his feet.

"Do you read much, Marcus?" I ask while I start my first set of crunches.

"I read history," he says and looks away for a moment. "We have had revolutions in this country. Did you know that?"

"I did." I can't tell how far he will go with this conversation.

"We have had bad times when the schools closed and the students were sent down to the fields," Marcus says quietly. "They worked with the peasants. Or they joined the army. Very hard times. You should read our history books and write about it to tell your country."

"I would like that," I say. Is he joking? Me write a new version of Chinese history? But—this is the thing that always catches me about Marcus—he is completely sincere. I'm sweating now. I'm waiting for him to say I can get off this machine. "But I think it would be too difficult."

"It would be very hard for you." He nods. "So much to learn. I had a professor in college." Marcus smiles now. "He was a historian. He was smart. I was too busy playing sports in college. I could never stay in the classroom. This professor, he said that if you were born after 1980 in China, then you had no past. You were the young generation and the hard times were over."

"Is this true?" I ask, panting.

"Oh, it is very true. The young people here, they care only for their video games and movies. They do not read. My college professor, he also said something else. He told me that if you were born before 1976 in China, then you had no future."

"Because you were too old?"

"Because you had lived through the hard times. But you would never adjust. You would always be living in the past. Okay, another round." He motions to the abs crunch bench. "One, two, three, let's go." I begin a new round of twenty. "Mao was the leader of the revolution," Marcus says. "Did you know that our old people starved? That the ones alive today have gone many days in their lives without eating?"

"I have heard that," I say. We are alone in the corner of the gym. I am fairly certain no one can hear us, unless the gym is bugged, which is never out of the question. But why is he talking about this today? I cannot figure out a way to tell Marcus that in our country we know about Mao—that our government uses the Great Leap Forward and the Cultural Revolution as examples of everything that's wrong with Communism.

"We do not understand that kind of mass hunger in my country," I explain. "We have had hard times. Years of trouble. We've had civil war and the Great Depression of the 1930s. Did you hear about this time?"

"The great what?"

"We call it the Great Depression. Many people lost their jobs. This was one time in our country when many people were hungry and starved."

"But it was your economy that was the problem. Right? Not your leaders?" Marcus stands back and stretches his neck from side to side. I wonder if he's nervous. "In China, it's the people who are the problem. The politicians. They are the ones who cause the suffering."

We move on to a leg press machine. Marcus keeps forgetting how many sets I've done and makes me do five instead of three. "There was a movie in 1994," he says and counts my repetitions in Chinese. "It was the first American film to change the way the Chinese saw Americans. Do you know it? It was called *For Gun*."

"Huh?" I say and stop. My thighs are burning. The hip-hop music is blasting. "I do not know this movie."

"Tom Hanks was the actor. It was a huge movie here."

"I think you mean *Top Gun*."

"Yes, yes, that's it. With Tom Hanks. *For Gun*."

I study Marcus's lips. "No, that's *Top Gun*," I say. "I think you mean *Top Gun*. Tom Cruise was in *Top Gun*." It's always alarming to hear what movies the Chinese have watched to form their impressions of America. Often it's Sylvester Stallone or Arnold Schwarzenegger films. I can't get my mind around the idea of the rest of the world misreading our nation based on the *Terminator* series.

"I am sure it was Tom Hanks." Marcus looks away. "I remember now: *Forest Gun* was the name."

"Oh, you mean *Forrest Gump*." I climb off the machine.

"Yes. Yes. *Forrest Gump* was the first time we saw an American movie in China that was not about killing or war. It was the first time we understood that Americans were more interesting. It was when we began to understand America. We did not have the Internet then. We only had government-censored TV. We did not know what Americans looked like. Now we understand. Now everyone is on the Internet."

I nod at him. Better *Forrest Gump* than *Top Gun*.

"We do stretching now," Marcus says and points. "Come." Stretching means I sit down on a weight bench and Marcus lifts both my hands over my head. Then he pulls on my elbows and shoulders until my arms dangle loose like chicken bones. I have to breathe in and out and close my eyes because it hurts on the side of the surgery. "You are stronger now," he says when he's finished. "Your form is better. You look better too. Much better than when we started."

# Office Party

The next night I have to decide what to wear to Tony's office party. It's a slapdash thing, he told me yesterday. There's no funding for parties like this now that the economic sky has fallen. But Tony says you still have to get together—you still have to try to build morale. I agree. I just wish the morale-building didn't have to involve me. I don't go out much these days. But Tony says many spouses have agreed to come—the Chinese husbands and wives of the software engineers and consultants who work in Tony's office.

I choose a green-flowered wraparound dress from my closet. It sounds bad but it's actually fine with the high black boots I wear it with. I look normal in this dress, and by that I mean that my breasts look normal. Which is always my goal now. In this dress the fake one on the left sits almost directly parallel to the real one on the right.

The party is set up with five long banquet tables and boiling pots of broth at each place setting. Someone has put large plastic bottles of Coke and Sprite in the middle of each table. Wine is not a Chinese custom at dinners like this. But soon, waiters bring out warm bottles of Yanjing beer. Tony wants people to mingle before they sit down. He tells me he hates it when everyone in the office runs for their seats. The music

helps. Tony hired a Brazilian singer from our apartment building named Lucio, who sings "The Girl from Ipanema." But
everyone still seems uncomfortable. They are awkward—as
if they don't know how to make small talk with their cubicle
partners. As if they've never done this before. "Why don't
they want to mix it up?" Tony asks me.

I tell him he's trying to make a Chinese office party into
an American cocktail hour. And it kind of works. But only
because Tony and Eric, Tony's second in command, fan out
around the room. "We won't be eating for at least an hour," I
hear Tony say to many of the men. "Come listen to the music.
No need to sit. No need."

The next time I'm near Tony, he is standing beside Lucio's
electric piano, going over a small list his Chinese office manager, Cynthia, has made of the order of events. That is when
he looks at me and says, "I tried to keep you out of it. I really
tried."

I'm drinking my second glass of Sprite and pretending it is
Sauvignon Blanc. I have no idea what he means. I'm hoping
we can sit down soon. I'm hoping this night will pass quickly.
If I'm honest, I'm hoping this whole year will pass quickly.
Because on the calendar I keep in my head, each year that
passes takes me further away from the cancer.

"Right," I say to him. "I'm just here to listen and support
you." It's important to him that I've come to the party. For
a short while, when we first returned to Beijing, I thought I
needed to distance myself from everyone, even Tony, in order
to get better. I think I was trying to isolate the disease. Isolate
myself. I can see now that this was not the best way.

"And that's why"—Tony tries to smile—"when they call
your name, just stand up quickly and come to the microphone
and I'll take it from there."

"They're not going to call my name," I whisper loudly in

his ear. "Because I am not going up to the microphone. That's not why I came. Remember. Not at all why I came."

"Oh yes you are." Tony smiles. "You have no choice. Cynthia has gotten you a gift."

"Oh God."

"Oh yes. And there's more."

"There can't be."

"There are games. Marriage games."

"I'm going to sit down now," I say. "I'm not listening to you anymore."


The gift Cynthia hands me up at the microphone is a cut-glass fruit bowl with red psychedelic swirls running through it. She has a glass bowl for each of the other six wives at the party, who are forced to listen to their husbands give short, painfully awkward speeches about how grateful the men are for spousal devotion. Cynthia has talked the men into doing it, and it's a kind of public praise that doesn't seem to come naturally here. I wince while the wives stand on the stage and look down at the ground.

At least Tony is able to skip the devotion part. When it's my turn to receive a bowl, he takes the microphone and says, "Susan and I would like to thank all of you for your hard work this year and for your support. We don't know many people here in China, and you have been like family to us." I smile and clap when the audience claps and think that these people have not really been like family. At least not to me. I hardly ever see these people. But it occurs to me that they might be like Tony's family—his extended Chinese family. How lucky for him. A part of me is jealous. How different Tony's and my days look in Beijing. He spends his time in an office with these interesting colleagues and gets to speak Chinese all day. I'm proud of him for what he's done here—brought the company to China. Forged relationships.

I go sit down with my fruit bowl, but Cynthia calls me back. She says into the microphone that the games are beginning and asks me to take a seat onstage. Then she waves the other six wives up and gives them seats too, and blindfolds. No one said anything about blindfolds. The object of the game, Cynthia announces, is for the seven husbands, also blindfolded, to take each woman's hand and figure out which is their wife.

My chair is first in the row. When the game begins, a strange man takes my fingers in his sweaty palm. "Is she your wife?" Cynthia asks him.

He presses my hand with his thumb and says with confidence, "Yes. This is my wife." Which produces squeals from the audience. My new husband and I are herded off to the side in our blindfolds, where we wait, hand in hand, while the rest of the group tries to mate.

When it's Tony's turn, I hear him walk down the row of seated women with outstretched hands, quickly saying to each one, "No, not my wife. Not my wife. None of these is my wife."

In the end, he's paired with Jenny, the shy office secretary. When they stand together and hold hands, the audience cannot contain itself. People snort with laughter, they're having so much fun. I smile and smile and think that if I have to smile any more my face will freeze. The finale comes when everyone takes off their blindfolds—all fourteen of us—and we realize that not one husband was able to find his own wife.

And even though I'm standing in front of a crowd of strangers, paired with a man I believe is married to Sophie Wu, the new office translator, I am still moved by my husband's show of loyalty. By his knowingness of me, and that he did not mistake me for someone else.

When we're allowed to go back to our table, I slink down low in my seat and guzzle more Sprite. That's when Alan, in presales, gets up and takes the microphone. He smiles and, with no warning, begins belting out a Frank Sinatra song: "My Way."

This is not on Cynthia's schedule. We all stare, and then the audience begins to clap and cheer. They love the song. People are warming up now. They seem to think the singing is a fantastic end to an amazing night. Alan is earnest and off-key, and I begin to laugh silently, and then the laughing turns into giggling until I'm not quite able to get a handle on it. I bite the insides of my cheeks hard and bend down to pretend to fix my shoe. This is no time to unravel.

The singing is infectious. Now Frank stands up. The crowd cheers when he says he's going to do a traditional folk song from his home province of Hebei. He begins, and it sounds like he's screaming: high-pitched, loud, Chinese screaming. He opens his mouth unnaturally wide to get the sounds out. We can see his molars. The audience begs for more. When are we ever going to go home? Tony has family here now. My people are thousands of miles away, in cities where it is either too late or early to call because of the baffling time change.

Frank does another folk number, and just when it looks like Eric is going to take the stage to sing, Tony jumps up and grabs the microphone. "Thank you, Frank," Tony says in Chinese, and smiles. "Thank you for that treat."

# Rose

I saw Rose again today. It's almost spring in Beijing, and we met for tea on the indoor porch of a café called The Face. There were red antique tea tables. We sat on a pink-flowered couch. She looked older. Rounder. Her glasses frames are green now. She wore jeans. She always wears jeans. And this time a small fitted gray cape over a T-shirt. We ordered mango puer tea and snacks. She brought presents for the boys: Chinese picture books. She kept laughing her wonderful, high-pitched laugh.

"Are there a lot of Chinese people going to Turkey?" I wanted to know.

"Medium amount of people," she said. "But more soon if Turkey joins the EU, because Chinese people see it as a way to get to Spain or Italy."

"Do you like the job?" I asked. "Do you like it more than teaching?"

"I like the fixed salary. I make four thousand yuan a month, but it is constant. When I taught, sometimes I made two thousand. Sometimes six thousand. But it was never steady, and I was always tired."

A waitress brings two pots of tea and then three stacked trays of bite-sized food. Rose unwraps the fork and knife from the paper napkin. She asks me how she is supposed to use the fork. "Do I hold it in my right hand or my left?"

"It's complicated," I say and show her. "You cut with the knife in your right hand, and then you switch it back. Or you can just leave your fork in your left hand. That's okay too." There are small ham sandwiches on toasted bread, and tuna with lettuce on miniature croissants. The tuna is surprisingly good. "How is your boyfriend?" I can't help but ask.

"He is out of a job. My parents came for the Chinese New Year and said they did not want to see him. They think he is a nice boy, but he is not the one for me to marry. So I told him I was going home, when really I stayed here the whole time with my parents."

"This sounds complicated. This sounds hard. Did he ever suspect you were still here?"

"I did a very good job of tricking him."

"Both your parents came?"

"They stayed in my apartment. They like my new place. It is very nice." Rose looks tired to me.

"What are your work hours?"

"It is not so bad. Eight hours a day and a half hour for lunch. But there is pressure." She takes off her glasses. "There is so much pressure."

"Do you mean from your boss?" I bite into a lemon tart.

"My boss is a Turkish official. She rejects most of the visa applications. Even the ones I approve. She has final say. She cannot read Chinese. Or speak it. I have to write my reports in English." Rose claps her hands in delight. "This is a very good thing! This helps me practice. And I can tell that most of the applicants are faking it."

"What do you mean, faking it?"

"The people are poor peasants from the countryside, but they come to the visa office pretending to be businessmen.

They create false stories of companies they run and colleagues. Then I call the company and I can tell it's not a real boss on the line—they're speaking with an accent that's wrong for the province. I call the wife listed on the application and I can tell she's not the real wife, because she doesn't know the name of her husband right away."

"Wow," I say, and take a sip of tea.

She smiles. "I used to be nice to the people. People would get their visas rejected but they would not leave the visa office. They would keep coming to my desk and asking me why. At first I tried to be helpful. I did not know any other way. Then one day last fall, a colleague told me I was too nice. He approached me during the working hours. He said, 'We are not a hotel. We are not a restaurant. You are not offering a service. You are being too good to these people. You have authority now. You need to demand respect.' And so I got a little meaner. I changed."

I thought I could see this in her face—it was harder now. And her eyes did not sparkle as much. I wanted to say, "Don't change! Don't change." She told me of a kind old Chinese couple who came to the office with an application because they wanted to go see their son and grandson in Turkey. "They had the right paperwork. They had money saved. I approved them. Because everything about them was appropriate. But my boss turned them down. The only reason she gave was that they were old. She said she was certain they would want to stay and live in Istanbul. I had to tell the couple. They did not understand. I had to ask them to leave my desk in the end."

We finish our tea. I'm trying to connect the Rose at the visa office to the Rose who taught me how to say "Hello, how are you?" in Chinese. There is some distance to travel between the two.

We walk out to the street. Rose asks me if I would like

to play mahjong with her girlfriends sometime next month. "Just girls," she says. "I want you to meet my friends."

"Sounds great," I say. "Sounds really good." I am not sure if we will see each other again. If I will ever meet her friends. Our connection in this teeming city seems fleeting to me now. Rose is not my Chinese teacher anymore.

"You have homework, Susan." Rose smiles. "You must learn to read the Chinese characters for the numbers one through ten. Each character. If you do this, then you will be able to play mahjong with me." Then she opens the cab door, steps inside, and is gone.

# Glitter

It's Saturday night and Tony and I revive the lost tradition of date night. Aidan is eating yogurt from a mug on the floor while he watches his brother dance naked to the Jackson Five. The song is "ABC." Mao Ayi watches from the kitchen door. She's going to babysit for us tonight. I'm waiting for Tony to get out of the shower so we can go. The music is cranked and Thorne jumps up on the couch. Mao Ayi is laughing now and moving her body. Then she starts taking small steps: 1-2-3, 1-2-3. It's the ballroom dancing I've seen all over China.

Aidan calls out to his brother, "I think this is a song about love."

Thorne yells back, "Maybe Michael wants a girlfriend. Because his brothers all have one." Thorne keeps leaping from the couch to the rug and screaming in the song whenever Michael does.

"He's the youngest one," Aidan reminds us. "Michael is the youngest and he hasn't made a girlfriend yet."

Tony and I say good-bye and take a cab to a Japanese sake bar called Manzo down a crowded alley on the other side of Chaoyang Park. The tables are white and the blue plates have tiny fish painted on them. Billie Holiday plays on the sound system. The Chinese waitress brings us a small chalkboard of handwritten fish specials. We order shrimp and grilled squid and cold Asahi beer from the tap.

I toast Tony for his month, for his year, for creating an office for his company here out of nothing. I toast him for his grace under pressure, and I mean it. He has an ease in China now.

He toasts me too. We're not big on toasts, but he says he's happy to sit here with me and eat the fish and drink the beer. He predicts we will have many good years to come. And this is just like him—to think of our future and not our past. I'm grateful to Tony for that too, for moving us forward.


When I was in college I lived with a boyfriend from Canada. When he graduated, he hung on in our Vermont town waiting for me to finish school. We were the couple who could never decide if we were meant to be together. We both wanted to be writers. One day I opened his journal while he was working as a sous-chef at the local inn. It was a deceitful thing to do. He always left it on the bedside table. Inside, he'd started a letter to a friend he'd been in a rock band with. It said, "I'm living with a girl who is too attached to the past."

I read his words, and then I put the journal down like it was burning. What did it mean? To be attached to the past? I knew I was implicated. Somehow his sentence sounded like a code for something much worse than nostalgia. After I graduated, he and I packed our things and drove to Toronto. We talked about marriage. He was a funny, brilliant person. But I always carried his words in my head. And he was probably right. I *was* attached to the past. I didn't know then how that would translate in my life. Or if it was really a bad thing in the end. I always wanted to tell him I'd read the letter. But I never did. And then we both married other people.

Sometimes, during my cancer treatment, Tony has served as the gatekeeper to my past. He's always up for the next doctor's visit, the next surgery. He sees no worth in revisiting history. He doesn't like me to dwell on yesterday or the day before. This is a sticking point for us. Because sometimes I think the past holds clues. On certain bad days I can't help myself—I relive the last few years or months, trying to detect a crack. Trying to deduce where the cancer might have crept in. Tony catches me in the act and says *What matters is that you're healthy. Why all the looking back?*

After dinner, Tony and I take another cab to The Hotel G, where the bar is retrofitted in raw slabs of concrete. There's a speed-dating party going on. The Chinese organizer asks if we want to join. "Even though you are married," she says in English, "you can just do it to meet people."

So we find ourselves sidled up to the bar—surely the only married couple there—with singles filling out white information sheets about themselves with small pencils. I would guess the male to female ratio is two to one. Lots of smokers. The average age is thirty. A man to my right is wearing something around his neck that looks like a cross between a tie and a scarf. There's a DJ spinning vinyl near the far window, and the electronica he plays has a heavy backbeat, with fake clapping and a synthesizer that simulates the sounds of laser guns.

Tony and I order single-malt whiskeys—something to sip while we watch. Most of the men lean their backs against the bar. Many of the women wear black dresses. The blender does not stop whirring fruit-flavored drinks. A lot of the speed-daters get out their cell phones and pretend to be busy. A teenage Chinese boy wearing a lime green down parka walks into the bar and then walks out.

I think there might be a lot of lonely people in China. I've read that since parents no longer arrange the marriages, there's a new restlessness in the country. People keep trickling into the bar. The staff rushes to take drink orders. There's a Chinese man with a white teapot in front of him who has no one to talk to and keeps tapping the bar with his hand. The man with the scarf that looks like a tie approaches the bar and orders another beer. I can see green glitter sparkling on his face. The organizer runs over and tells us the dates will be in five-minute intervals. I want to sip my drink and watch, but Tony keeps egging me on.

"It will be fun," he says. "One of those once-in-a-lifetime things. You can write about it. Do research."

When I met Tony, I prepared for a life of triangulation: China, my husband, and me. But not tonight. It's late now. Mao Ayi must be wondering. I'm tired and I want to go home. *I am already married,* I turn and say to my husband. *To you. I am married to you.*

When we get to the apartment, Mao Ayi is waiting on the couch. She's had a busy night, she explains to Tony in Chinese. Both boys wanted *pai pai.* She says it took a long time to pai pai Aidan and then Thorne was mad because he'd been waiting for his pai pai.

"Pai pai" is what Mao Ayi calls patting the boys' backs while she sings them songs in bed. She loves to do it. The boys have gotten wise to what a good thing they have going. Because Mao Ayi will do pai pai *until* you have fallen asleep. Which is a lot longer than my American version of pai pai.

The boys discussed it in the afternoon before Tony and I went out—who would get it first and for how long. Thorne was jealous because last time, it took Mao Ayi so long to pai pai Aidan that Thorne fell asleep waiting and never got his. Mao Ayi stands up from the couch and goes to the hall to put on her leather jacket. She wears a proud smile and tells us again how the boys were crying—*They were fighting,* she says in Chinese, *over which one would get the first pai pai.*

# Chinese Basketball

It's the first day of March again—a warm Wednesday after-noon in Beijing—and I wait for the bus with the Taiwan-ese moms, who've just returned from another one of their long karaoke lunches. Flora's best friend, Judy, is there. She always has a smile for everyone. I ask her how her son is. "He is too short," Judy says with a serious face. "He is just too short and it's a big problem."

I have to give Judy credit for her candor. No one I know in the States would say what Judy has just said. Judy herself is one of the shortest people I've met in China. She says she doesn't understand why her son is so small and that she tells him every day to grow. "I get him to play basketball too. I think jumping will help him grow taller."

Judy asks me if I want to get in on a bulk order of sea-weed the Taiwanese moms are having shipped from the home country. "It's the best seaweed in the world," Judy says. "It has minerals and iron and calcium for growing bones." I order two packages and am supposed to pay her when the shipment comes in.

When Thorne gets off the school bus, he looks to me like he's of average height. I make a mental note to check on this soon. He announces that he is Villager Number Two in the school's Robin Hood musical. Back at the apartment, I look in his notebooks until I find the play's script and read it through. It turns out Villager Number Two has one line in the entire production. Count it. One. But Thorne's upbeat about it. He's the only second grader with a speaking part, and he has twelve songs to memorize, which means he walks through the apartment singing again. This time the songs are not patriotic, or sung out of some raw dislocation anxiety. *Robin. Robin Hood. Always doing good. He steals from the rich and gives to the poor.* I think Thorne's made it to the other side. Beijing is where he lives now. He's more like himself here than ever before. Or maybe he's changed into someone else entirely in China, someone he never would have become in Portland.

On Thursday I go to the school assembly because Thorne tells me he's reading a poem onstage. When it's time for the second graders, my son bounds up the three stairs to the microphone stand, where he recites a piece he's written in homeroom called "Mother." I had no idea this was coming. I wasn't sure if Thorne even liked me anymore—I'd been distracted so much of last year, tired and spacey from the surgery and the treatment. Thorne's poem has words in it like *loving* and *defending* and *awesome.* I sit frozen in my chair, tears leaking from my eyes, and I know this is one of the moments to pay attention to. They don't come crystallized like this often.

All year long I've hoped Thorne knew how much he mattered. Every week I asked him—*Do you know how much?* Even when he said *Yeah, yeah* and smiled, I wanted a better answer. Wanted to tell him again, just in case there came a time when I wasn't here to do it anymore.

Everyone claps when Thorne finishes his poem, but my cheering for him goes on much longer inside my head. It hasn't stopped, really. My eight-year-old is still not too cool for school. Who knew we would make it this far away from the specter of cancer? And that we'd be more or less intact? Or that Thorne would read a poem onstage in China and take a bow with a wide smile on his face?

An hour later Aidan gets up onstage too. Except he's wearing a shiny purple velour sweat suit the music teacher's put him in, and he's singing a Chinese song about an African crocodile. He has two maracas in his hands, and he shakes them to the beat. I'm crying again but it's because I'm laughing so hard. Not *at him*. Aidan would never forgive me for that. I'm laughing at how much fun it is to see him up there, singing his lungs out. What Aidan has done in China is to make it his home. It took a long time. He was not easily convinced.

The other things Aidan has done in China are to get taller and to learn how to read. The impact of both of these on him can't be understated: he's almost as tall as his brother now, and no one in our family owns the inside track on reading anymore. Aidan has friends here, too. Aidan likes deep connections—to mark his friends with an X and not let them go. He seems aware of the precariousness of it all. He likes to double-check. Just to be sure. When we got home after the concert today, there was a birthday invitation for him on my computer from his friend Liam. That party is Saturday. "There's four days between now and then," Aidan said, counting on his hand. "What if Liam changes his mind? Can he take back a party invitation once he's mailed it?"

. . .

One of the things I do now is talk to other women who've had breast cancer. The hospital back in Boston has set up an international phone line for us to call in to. And what an amazing thing that is. I'm in touch with six other women my age who are finishing their treatment. Great, funny women. We have a weekly phone call, and a therapist joins us. Talking to these women helps defuse the fear. There's so much to say. An entire new language opens up—there are words about the worry of it that I've been holding in. I say them into the phone, and they start to lose their power.

The other thing I do with my time is more yoga. I still have pain in my left shoulder and along my rib cage. I meet Mimi on Wednesday and she asks me to see if I can try not thinking for whole minutes at a time. She tells me to breathe instead of think—to let the front of my brain drop away until I feel myself settle into my body. I've been scared of my body since the surgeries, afraid of what I might find there. Mimi says, "Watch yourself relax while you stretch, and take joy in that."

Joy in it? How did she know there would be any joy left? I see how I've been ruminating on the cancer—still guilty of trying to solve for it. I haven't wanted to spend time with myself. I lie down on the mat and stare at the white ceiling and begin to be able to be thankful for what I still have. For my husband. My children. Even my health.

Today's yoga class ends with thirty minutes of Sanskrit chanting. I've never chanted before, but it's just another thing I try for the first time in China that feels out of my comfort zone. Mimi leads us in the chanting, and I can't get over the easiness of her voice—how it hits the high notes and then comes back down to earth. Everyone keeps their eyes closed the whole time we chant, and the feeling is one of being supported, propped up by the sound of so many other people's voices in the room. I don't feel so alone in China anymore.

After yoga I walk over to the Bookworm to listen in on a journalists' roundtable talk, and I'm calm in the way that chanting for thirty minutes in Sanskrit in the lotus position for the first time can make you. The room is packed, and we all have pens out and little notepads on our laps. It's just one week after the anniversary of last year's Tibetan protests, so expectations in the audience are high.

One journalist starts by announcing that all forms of print journalism will be dead in twenty years. And isn't that depressing. But we aren't here to talk about that. We want to know what it's like to stand on the front lines in China. We're after *news*. We want the reporters to tell us if access will get better in China—if there's a way to uncover, as one person asks, "the real truth here." Which is another way of wondering how long this thing they call Communism will be around. I want that question answered in a hungry way.

How hard is it to cover a story in China? I want them to tell us that too. The *Los Angeles Times* reporter tells us that a *New York Times* reporter has just been released after being held for twenty hours in a room in Yunnan Province with no explanation. He'd been walking around Tibetan houses there looking for a protest story.

Then an American professor reminds us that in totalitarian regimes the people don't trust their government, and the government doesn't trust its own people. The one Chinese expert on the panel says the Communist Party puts up walls to keep information from getting out of China, but the Chinese people just put up higher ladders. "Western reporters need to hold China to the same standards they hold the rest of the world to. China wants the foreign press to be nice," he explains. But, he reminds us, "News is usually bad, because bad news is news." There are bright spots, he says, in China's understanding of free press. "For example, during the Olympics, the Chinese government had to attend press conferences and answer hard questions. Unfortunately"—he pauses—"the questions were only about the weather."

# Caskets

Yesterday was May 14, the one-year anniversary of my mastectomy, and I got stuck in our elevator. Elevators have always set me on high alert. They make me think of caskets. When I rang the alarm bell, nothing happened. Then I pressed the call button and began what I would call a long, heated exchange with some teenage security guard, who kept screaming at me in Mandarin. I believe he was asking me where I was. I believe I was telling him that I was on the eighth floor.

I should have assumed nothing. That is always a better way to proceed in Beijing. Assume nothing will unfold as planned and then everything is slightly surprising and more pleasant than predicted. "Wo yao yi ge ren!" *I want someone,* is what I screamed. (It was the only thing I could think of in Mandarin to say.) *I want someone.*

I got bitchy. I called Tony on his cell phone while he was in a very important meeting with Chinese bankers. I did not let him speak. I said, "No. No. I don't care where you are. I am stuck in the elevator and you have to get me out of here."

"Calm down," Tony said slowly, "and tell me exactly where you are."

"Stuck in the elevator. I already told you." My voice was rising.

"But where, Susan? Where are you?"

"In our apartment building, for God's sake. In Beijing. Where do you think I am?" I was in a boxing match with claustrophobia and I had to punch back or the feeling would trap me. Which is why I then said some pretty mean things to Tony. I felt like the elevator was getting smaller and smaller. "I AM IN CHINA," I yelled at him. "IN THIS GODFORSAKEN COUNTRY YOU HAVE BROUGHT US TO WHERE THEY DO NOT HAVE AN ELEVATOR RESPONSE SYSTEM. I HAVE BEEN IN HERE FOR OVER TWENTY MINUTES."

That's when Tony asked the other people in the meeting with him if he could have five minutes alone to handle a personal emergency. "Susan," I heard him say slowly into the phone. "You are screaming at me and you're not being fair and I'm hanging up now. I am hanging up so I can call the building's security."

"Oh great," I said. "Great! Now you're being mean to me while I am stuck in the elevator." What I didn't understand until then was why people who are having anxiety attacks often lash out at others around them. They say things they don't mean. But it feels good. Every time I yelled at Tony I got a little distance on the claustrophobia. My anger connected me to him.

"Hanging up now," Tony said again. He was mad. I could tell. "I am hanging up."

"Asshole," is what I said next. "You are an asshole." Which was completely unfair and yet felt utterly sensible to me; at this point everyone I knew who was not stuck inside the elevator with me was an asshole. I could not see then that sometimes having cancer is like being stuck inside an elevator. Nor could I understand why my anger seemed so large. Then I started crying—I saw my face scrunch up and the tears flow because the elevator was lined with mirrors. I sobbed and I repeated in the empty air, "You are an asshole for hanging up on me."

But Tony was gone by then. He was trying to talk in Mandarin to the Park Avenue security managers—trying to get someone to run over to Tower Five and open up the elevator doors. Until Tony reached the management office by phone, no one on site knew I was stuck. No one had understood my Chinglish into the elevator's emergency sound system. They didn't have anyone speaking English to help.

I am embarrassed that I called my husband an asshole. He did not deserve it. But when he called me back and told me to sit tight—that someone would be there soon to let me out—I yelled at him some more about how today was the one-year anniversary of my mastectomy surgery and why hadn't he said anything about it to me? Which gets me back to the fact that most people, even the people who love me most dearly, don't always know how to talk about cancer.

Tony offered that his mind had been on my mastectomy all day. I said it didn't count just to think thoughts inside your head. You had to *voice* them. That was the key part of being a cancer patient for me. *People had to tell me what they were thinking about the cancer.* If not all of it, then at least the good parts. And if they didn't have anything good to say, then they should make something up. "Saying what you think is part of our marriage," I yelled into the phone at Tony. "It's how we are able to stay in China," I reminded him. "We have to say the things we're thinking."

Then I heard a call waiting beep. I was sweating by then

and feeling nauseous. I wondered if the claustrophobia would make me throw up or faint. Everything felt like a crisis. The call was from Aidan and Thorne's school bus ayi, asking me where I was because the bus had been waiting ten minutes. "I can't come," I said to her in English. "I'm stuck in an elevator." I have no idea how much of that sentence the Chinese bus monitor understood.

Tony called me back and said, "I know you're hurting. I know you're scared. I know it's a terrible anniversary so I'm going to forgive you for what you said."

"I need you to call Mao Ayi," is how I answered him. I had no interest in his forgiveness. I wanted more of his attention. I needed all of it. "Call Mao Ayi and tell her she needs to run down the eight flights of stairs to go get Aidey and Thorne." What I wanted to tell him was he had *no idea* what it's like to have a mastectomy or to be stuck in a high-rise Chinese elevator for twenty-five minutes with no sign of help. But in the end, I didn't tell him either of those things. Instead, what I did was get quiet. I realized that the yelling was only working me up more.

Then I heard an older Chinese voice on the elevator speaker: "It is me." *Who?* I wanted to ask. He said, "I am sorry. It is my fault that you are stuck in the elevator. Can you please wait five more minutes?"

I didn't know what to say, so I said, "Okay." I said, "Fine." And then I recognized the voice—not the actual person behind the voice, but the voice itself. It was the voice of Chinese civic responsibility. It was the voice of communal duty—the one that takes the collective blame. Because in Beijing, so much still depends on the Confucius way: the hierarchical order. The acceptance of consequences.

A small man in a blue utility uniform finally opened

the elevator doors. He held what looked like a crowbar in his hands. Six people stood behind him: property managers and sub-managers in blue and white Park Avenue uniforms. All of them stared at me while the doors slowly parted. For one second I felt like a trapped animal set free. But I was not done yet with my anger. I stepped off the elevator and I screamed at them. I said that my sons had been waiting for me on their school bus. I said it was terrible that they didn't have one single person in the elevator control room who spoke English. I yelled at the people and they stared back at me silently. One of them could have reminded me that I was in *their country*. And that I could have gotten myself together and learned some more Chinese—at least the words for *trapped in the elevator*. But these people were too polite to tell me to get off my high horse. They stared at me and nodded. Then I slammed my apartment door shut and began crying again. What I think I meant to say was that mastectomies lingered, and so did anniversaries of mastectomies. It's a date I should lose track of.

# Tiger Leaping Gorge

Those are my two boys up ahead on the horses. Aidan is riding the brown one named Huami. Thorne straddles the paler one, Haley. Both boys think their Chinese horses are the greatest animals in Asia. Maybe in the world. We are in a steep mountain gorge in southern Yunnan Province during May Chinese Holiday Week. There's also a guide named Aki with us. He has a long black ponytail and comes from a minority tribe near here called the Yi. Aki explains to me while we walk that his people used to be bandits who came down from the mountains at night and kidnapped Han townspeople as slaves.

The land here is a spectacular shade of bright green with terraced cornfields and rectangular rice paddies and acres of sunflowers. The peak of Tiger Leaping Gorge is over ten thousand feet high, and the path we're on snakes the side of the mountain. Sometimes the drop is too high for me to look, and I hug the cliff and wonder. But mostly I feel calm. Aidan could ride Huami for eight hours each day and not want to get off. Both boys smile at me whenever I run and catch up with them. Aki has taught them to lean forward into their horses' necks when they go up hills, and to lie back in the saddle on the way down.

After two hours of climbing, we stop at the home of Lao Du, the owner of the horses. His house is made of clay and brick. It has no electricity or running water and overlooks a deep V the river cuts between the stone mountainsides. Two wooden chairs with torn upholstery sit on the brick stoop. Lao Du's wife motions to one of the chairs and gives me a cup of mint tea and two Chinese pears. She is a tiny woman wearing a Levi's jean jacket in the heat. When she smiles, which is often, her whole face lights up. She hands Tony a bowl of walnuts and a round stone to crack them with.

We are miles from the nearest town, and there is a small convenience store on one side of the Dus' porch: a red freezer hooked up to a generator contains Popsicles and ice cream bars. Crackers and potato chips and batteries are also for sale. Aidan chooses a pineapple Popsicle. Thorne takes a mango one.

Aki tells Tony that the Dus have lived on this land for centuries. He says that all the money they make goes to keeping their son and daughter in school. There is no school in the mountains, and their children board down in the nearest city. We eat the fruit and nuts and Popsicles and then stand and thank the Dus for their kindness. On the way out, we pass their neighbor—an older, stouter woman who sits on her own porch and does not smile at us. She has what looks like a competing convenience store: stacks of Wrigley's gum, a glass fridge full of Cokes and Sprites. She turns and glares as we walk by.

I have just begun to consider forgiving everyone in my life who does not have breast cancer. This is no small thing. There is still a part of me that wants to hold something against healthy people. Not for being healthy—not for that exactly. My resentment has to do with an essential aloneness that cancer has woven into my days.

Here in Yunnan, the mountaintops stack one behind the other and create the illusion of stretching high into the ancient Chinese heavens. Many of the sunflower crops that line the path have blossomed into a swath of yellow. Tony is happy to be here. He's got this reckless look in his eye that signals his willingness to live in Tiger Leaping Gorge for the rest of our lives. Soon I bet he'll start talking about home schooling the boys and inquire about farmhouse rentals in the valley. Meanwhile he's taking hundreds of pictures of the mountains and the boys on their horses. "They love it here, don't they?" he says as he squeezes by me on the path on his way to catch up with Aidan and Huami. "I knew the boys would love Yunnan. And you too—you love Yunnan, don't you? I knew you would." I don't have to answer him when he gets like this. I just smile, and that's enough to convince him.

I do like it here. Everything in the gorge has turned an even brighter green from recent rains; the wild grasses and evergreen trees, corn stalks and rice plants are full and lush and appear to ripple down to the river, which lies almost out of sight. We stop for the night in a scattering of houses built into the side of the mountain. I sit in the stone courtyard of the guesthouse and cannot get enough of the view.

Dinner is round loaves of warm bread served with sliced chicken or apples and bananas on top. Tony asks Aki if farmers in the valley make money off their crops. Aki stares into the distance and then says, "The farmers in Yunnan are very angry. The corruption makes them furious."

"Is everyone in town corrupt?" Tony bites into the bread.

"A farmer cannot get the right price." Aki points down the hill at a pear tree orchard. "Even in this tiny village there's a head man, and if you won't bribe him, you'll never see a profit on your pears. You'll never prosper. The corruption is so bad here you do not understand. You cannot get away from it. It is impossible."

"A by-product of socialism," I say.

"You cannot call this socialism," Aki corrects me. "That is a bad joke. That is a lie. This is capitalism. And if things do not change"—here Aki's face became serious—"in ten years it will be very dangerous in China."

In the morning, we climb down from the mountains with the horses until we're flush with the black river. It looks smaller now that we are closer to it, but still dangerous with its silent current. Aki has hired a van to take us to a Tibetan temple in the woods. The heavy rains have washed out the road in places, and we get stuck miles down a neglected stretch along a small lake. We climb out to look at the wheels sunk in brown mud. Aki disappears over the hill and comes back carrying tree branches, which he wedges under the tires. Four old Chinese men sit on their heels, smoking cigarettes up the hill, watching the free entertainment.

The driver guns the engine and tries to make the crest, but misses and slides down sideways, closer to the edge each time. The boys and I have been instructed to lie on top of the backpacks in the rear of the van to try to weigh things down. This feels unsafe. The lake is right below. Just when I'm thinking of climbing out, Aki and Tony push the van over the top of the hill, and we jump down and cheer and clap and high-five. We're closer to one another now than we were before the van got stuck. We drive without stopping through the mud across a stretch of wet field and up to a slightly higher dirt road until we get to the monastery.

Teenage monks greet us in the driveway in long maroon robes and flip-flops. They lead us to the front stairs, where we bow to a large Buddha statue. Aki explains that Chinese police guarded this monastery for weeks during the Tibetan protests last March. "Every day," he says, "police made a show of force over Yunnan. This is how the government was able to prevent protests in Yunnan while most other Tibetan towns were under siege."

Then he points to the young monks who sit along the sides of the courtyard kicking dirt. They look to be Thorne's age. "These boys," Aki explains, "are not learning math or science or history here. They are studying Buddhist texts. This is the real Tibetan problem. A problem of education."

The temple is well maintained, with dark rugs on the floors and bright blue and yellow paintings of bodhisattvas on the walls. I find Thorne and Aidan down on their knees in one of the smaller temples, praying in front of an ornate wooden altar. Aidan stands up first and runs to tell me he's prayed for the video game Wii and for our family to be healthy. Then Thorne says he prayed for the exact same thing, plus for his grandmothers.

Then it's my turn. I am not practiced. I thought I needed time for my thoughts to coalesce before I could get down on my knees again. I thought if I could only think on the disease a bit longer—a few more weeks to discern and deduce the cancer—maybe then I'd have the answers. I have probably thought too much. I kneel down and light one of the purple sticks of incense Thorne bought from the teenage monks.

I whisper out loud to the Buddha that I do not want these boys of mine to be motherless. "These boys right here," I say and point with my hand. "The ones who look so carefree." It's easier than I thought to surrender like this. There's an urgency to my prayer now: the tears run. I ask the Buddha to spare Thorne and Aidan. To somehow spare all four of us.

When I stand up, both boys are trying to balance on one leg by the open door. They are calm, almost reverent—as if they understand that something larger is at work in the temple. "What religion are we?" Thorne asks me eagerly. He's learned enough about Buddhism today to sign on. I can tell he likes being inside the temple with the monks moving around us. "Because I want to be Buddhist," he says. "I want to believe in reincarnation."

Aki finds us standing in the small room and Aidan asks him what his religion is. Aki says, "My tribe believes in family spirits. After I die, I will go meet the souls of my ancestors."

Aidan takes in Aki's words and then announces, "That's what I want to be. That religion. That one."

All year long the boys have been asking me what I believe in, and I've been able to avoid a full answer. I smile at them and reach out my hands to touch their heads. The next time they ask, I'll be better prepared. I'll explain to them that I have a new kind of faith now. A trustingness. And maybe it's passed down from a god, or gleaned from the earth. I'll say too that I believe in language. Thorne will probably counter that language is not a god—that words can't be my religion. I'll say, *Why not?* Because I've come to see that words are what get me up in the morning. What allow me to go down on my knees in this small temple and pray. Maybe in the end, words are something we can carry with us. Because the stories of our lives live on. And I would like my story to be about hope. It will also have the word *disease* in it, but that won't be my whole story.

. . .

We drive farther in the van and stop at a roadside canteen for lunch. Garbage is heaped outside the door and flies buzz around a coal-blackened ceiling. The boys and I count tires everywhere in the street—over fifty of them—and more piles of stray car parts. Tony laughs when I make a frown face and orders us boiled noodles with steamed bok choy. He says the towns in Yunnan are often organized like this: one village just for cars, one for woodworking, one for slippers. One for baskets.

We make it to a small town called Shaxi for the night. It is a slipper village. Fifteen sewing shops line the main street selling the same embroidered pink velvet shoes, or silk ones if you want, or traditional black ones for men. Who is going to buy all these? We sleep in a guesthouse called a caravan that is hundreds of years old—a place that used to lie on the Burma tea trail. Horsemen slept in these dark rooms and tied up their animals in the dirt plaza outside. Our room has white clay walls, with a floor made of hard dirt. We wake when the first person in the caravan stirs. I decide that no one in the Chinese countryside really sleeps. There is so much activity before the sun rises—so much clearing of the throat and spitting and checking on the chickens and pigs.

In the morning, Tony and I take the boys behind town to the rice fields. Rural China turns out to be a lesson in animal husbandry. A herd of white goats passes on the narrow footbridge, then six oxen. We watch a local woman from the Naxi tribe in a blue apron shoo one black pig past the paddies toward town. A man follows behind her with a loud flock of turkeys. He tells the boys in Chinese that we can come and talk to the turkeys whenever we want. I count seven horses on our walk back into the village. One mother donkey is tied to a tree while her foal is allowed to roam.

We take another path out of town and climb a hill to where a widower lives. He tells Tony it's his job to take care of the clear pond that sits next to his house. It is the village's only water source. The man invites us inside. There is a single wooden bed in the corner and a coal stove closer to the door. The ceiling above the stove is black. The man says he's been living there as long as he can remember and that his wife is dead now.

I go outside and listen to the sound of water from the mountains feed into the pond. The man tells the boys they can find minnows and freshwater crabs along the banks. I reject the notion of Tony as widower. He's only spoken of it to me once, when I was upset early on after the diagnosis and unable to sleep. He wanted me to know somehow that he understood my pain. And to see how far his pain had also gone. What he said helped, but it also scared me, and I think we've put that conversation away for good.

We walk down to the rice fields and balance on the small ridges above the muck and water. It rains again and our pace slows. Each of us falls into a paddy—Tony up to his thighs, me just to my knees. Once Aidan slips over the side of a steep edge, and we lose him for a second, then Aki laughs and hauls him back up. Tony tries to toss Thorne over a wide stream that splits the path in two, but Thorne lands on his back and yells, then I run over to him and hold him in my lap on the ground.

I can say that cancer has brought me closer to the boys. The disease distracted me from them at first. It called for all my attention, and that was alarming—that something could have a stronger claim on me than my children. Now there's a balancing out. It might be a purer kind of love I feel for them. This is partly because my love does not have as many requirements. I don't ask for as much back.

Or even wish for it. But I can also be further away from the boys now too, if this makes sense. More remote when I'm worried about dying before they're grown, or when I'm watching them—wondering what their lives would be like without me. This is one of the contradictions of illness: intimacy and distance with the people I love. It's something I do not talk about often, even with Tony. It's too confusing.

Thorne stands up from the ground and steps on a dead snake. When I was growing up in the woods in Maine, nothing scared me more than snakes. I like to believe nothing will scare me again, and that my boys are steady like their father. I've tried to make sure of that. I don't ever want my undoing to be theirs. I close my eyes and hold Tony's hand, and he guides me past the dead snake. A man stands in the field shaving a piece of wood with a long knife. He reaches out and touches Thorne's head and tells Tony he's never seen a foreign boy before.

I count the months we have left in China. By my calculations there are seven. Tony and I have decided this week that we'll move home next January. By then he'll have handed off the office baton to someone local, as planned. In a way this Yunnan trip marks the beginning of our China leave-taking. Part of me wants to go home—the part of me that's tired of bad air and permits and doctors who don't listen. But there's also another part—almost equally large—that would like to never go home.

China has proven to be the greatest road trip. And the thing about road trips is that they absolve you. Force you to give up control. They allow you to gaze out the window for hours at a time and fiddle with the radio dial and free you of most responsibilities except procuring decent snack food. I don't want this one to end.

We walk to another village beyond the rice fields. A slogan written on the wall of a farmhouse reads "Socialism is great." Aki reads this out loud and says it's just another Chinese lie. Then we slowly make it back to the caravan. Aidan and Thorne play soccer in the town square. A few local kids join until there's a full game. Three Chinese women in their fifties stop to play too. They laugh and kick the ball with the children until a man comes out of a store doorway and announces that everyone has to stop. He tells Tony it's too dangerous for other tourists to have a soccer game like this. I want to point out that we're the only tourists—Tony and Aidan and Thorne and me. There are no others I can see. Besides, I want to say, the locals like the game, and it doesn't seem to me like there's a lot else to do in town. Most of the kids tend to sit on the stoops of the slipper shops and stare out at the street.

But the players scatter, and the man retreats. Then one of the older women who'd been kicking the ball with Thorne approaches Tony and me and says in Chinese, "We are good listeners. But we love to play." She smiles at me and I grin back, happy that I can understand what she says. I'm more than willing to break the rules with her—we'll be okay. It's only soccer, after all. I reach my arms toward her. Then she picks the ball off the ground and throws it to me in the air.

# Houmen: The Back Gate

We left China on a gray, windy Wednesday in late December. The United flight to Chicago was scheduled to depart at 4:30 p.m. A team of teenage packers had stormed the apartment in the days before, leaving nothing in their wake; for ten hours they'd boxed and taped and stacked like maniacs. The bulk of our stuff—the boys' Chinese bikes and the calligraphy scrolls and a small collection of teapots—had been put on a slow boat due to arrive in New York City, we were told, some months down the line.

Things we needed sooner but couldn't fit in our duffels—down comforters, wool socks and hats, an enormous picture of the student body of the boys' school—were wrapped and placed in a wooden airfreight container meant to land in Portland the day we did. The movers worked so fast it was hard for Tony and me to keep up. I lost track of what was sea and what was air and if we would ever see any of this stuff again and why we had any of this crap anyway.

Lao Wu rang our doorbell at 10:00 a.m. He took off his loafers outside the elevator and walked into our long hall in his black ankle socks. We'd finally been able to talk him into coming up to our apartment. We'd cajoled him all week until he gave in. *Dumplings,* we'd said. *It's our last day*. He'd never wanted to come up before—always trying unsuccessfully to maintain the boundaries between work and friendship.

The apartment sat empty except for two last house-plants—a miniature fir tree we'd hung Christmas ornaments on, and a scrappy potted bougainvillea, both of which I planned to give to my new British friend, Claire. The turtles were still there, too—swimming in their glass bowl, impervious to our departure, still waiting to make a break. Mao Ayi had promised to adopt them. I'd tried several times that week to figure out how to ask her not to eat the turtles. I knew what a fondness the Chinese have for turtle soup, and it worried me the way she'd sometimes gaze longingly at them and measure their growth to me with her hands. "Hen da!" she'd called out to me the day before. *They are so big!*

Moving home was no longer a simple thing. Tony would have been happy to stay in Beijing. Sure, part of him was ready to go back to the States—and his contract was officially over. He'd handed off the baton and cleaned out his desk, and said he'd also tired of air thick as leek soup. But his patience for the country still seemed endless. The boys knew in theory we were moving home, and that sounded great to them. But so did going to a sleepover at Mads and Gustav's house on Saturday. And finishing the investigation of the speed of light at school, and practicing a song from the Chinese opera for the winter musical. The boys were in the thick of it—busy with the work of being first and third graders. What did they care about moving back to a country they had only vague memories of?

My reasons for returning were several. I wanted the boys to be able to walk to friends' houses again. We hardly ever walked anywhere in Beijing. I hoped their friends would move in and out of our house in a constant coming and going. Seeing friends in Beijing was a logistical quagmire of traffic and confusing Chinese addresses. But when I'm honest, I probably wanted to go back most for me.

I thought I needed to feel what it was like to be home again and healthy. Really home. It may make no sense, but I held on to the idea that by being back in our house I would once and for all be divested of cancer. I had never known cancer in that house, so maybe, just possibly, returning home would be like entering a small portal: we would be transported back to a time when we didn't know the data involved in cancer staging. When we hadn't learned the Chinese word for *disease*.

Lao Wu followed me into the kitchen—his stride was purposeful. He was here to do a job, and making the dumplings, we'd come to learn, is a big deal in China. An important part of almost every ritual. Thorne poked his head out of his bedroom, where I had him sorting the stuffed animals he wanted to bring in his backpack on the plane. He saw Lao Wu and ran down the hall to hug his waist. Then they did a little mock fighting pressed up against the dishwasher, yelling slights in Mandarin.

Mao Ayi put a stop to it. It was her kitchen, after all, and she was in charge. "Lai, lai," she yelled, and they both turned and walked over to her at the counter, where she put them to work. Aidan was already standing there on a dining room chair he'd dragged over. I leaned in the kitchen doorway watching while they pressed out dumpling dough with four wooden rolling pins. Then each of them began filling small pancakes of dough with Mao Ayi's mash of ground beef, green onion, cooked egg, and garlic.

Earlier that morning, just before she mixed the dumpling dough, Mao Ayi had called me into the front hall. "SOOZAN!" she yelled at the top of her lungs. "SOOO-ZAN!" I bolted out of Aidan's room, and there she was, standing next to a large blue and orange poster of the Buddha. There were three of them, actually—large-scale Buddhas, each one trippier and more psychedelic than the next: the Buddha in long, orange robes holding a lotus blossom while a deep electric yellow orb radiated from his crowned head. The Buddha shirtless in an orange sarong. The Buddha in blue with medallions around his neck. All three Buddhas appeared to be floating in black space.

"Ni xihuan ma?" Mao Ayi asked me eagerly. *Do you like it?* Then she told me she'd been worried that my little painting of the Buddha on my desk was just too small. "Tai xiao!" she said. *Not big enough.* I needed something more.

The poster reminded me of some bad 1970s heavy metal drug album—maybe Blue Oyster Cult or that British band named Yes. "Wo xihuan," I said, and smiled. *I like it.* How incredibly generous of her. How kind. And what in God's name was I going to do with it? The movers had come and gone. We'd been left with our eight overstuffed L.L.Bean duffels. We were almost out of there—almost gone from China, but not quite yet.

Tony got so excited by the dumpling making in the kitchen that he ran and grabbed his video camera. "I'm going to record each step!" he yelled to me from where he stood backed up against the refrigerator. "And then we can play it over and learn the recipe at home." I nodded and smiled at the scene and thought, *We can't leave China. We can't leave these kind people. We will never leave China.*

Then I went back to Aidan's room and tried to pack up his collection of rocks—an assortment of black and gray stones he's gathered all over the country. I put them in a plastic grocery bag. I sat on Aidan's rug and realized that the problem with leaving China was that Aidan and Thorne were happy here now. They chatted in Mandarin, and how could we leave the language behind? Another problem in leaving China was that in some ways Tony was the purest version of himself there—open and engaged and always curious, always hoping for the next train ride. China had called him out of his comfort zone and plunked him deep in that Daoist river.

I opened Aidan's sock drawer and found myself asking the same questions I'd voiced leaving Portland two and a half years ago: what would become of us in the move? I knew we'd been changed by China, but how exactly? Leaving meant we were closing a door. Marking time. In that way it was impossible to ignore that the four of us were all growing older.

Aidan's room looked beat-up—floorboards dinged from skateboarding and kick ball, white walls dirtied from smog and greasy fingers. It was hard to stand there and know that in a few short hours we'd be gone. That the apartment would sit empty—as if we'd never learned Chinese verbs there or sung compulsively or cried ourselves to sleep. I thought of how much living we'd done in those concrete rooms up above the Fourth Ring Road. Now we were leaving? How could we? How dare we?

Four days before our flight there'd been good-bye ceremonies for both boys at school. I'd sat in a small red plastic chair and watched while Thorne and Aidan climbed into inflatable rubber rafts in the middle of their classrooms. They played Handel's *Water Music* and then all of us stood up—the students and the boys' teachers and Julie, the principal, and me—and we swayed to the music. We were meant to imagine Thorne and Aidan riding in their rafts over the great expanse of the Pacific Ocean, headed home to the United States.

After the music finished, Aidan began reading a speech he'd crafted that morning: "I don't have the words to say how much I liked first grade." I held my camera over my eyes to hide my tears. He added for good measure that what he really looked forward to in America was going to a wood-oven pizza place he knew. "You sit on a stone bench," he told everyone, "and watch your own crust cook."

When Thorne spoke from his raft, he said he was grateful to his friends in third grade for making him "so comfortable here." I laughed and cried again for his word choice. Where was that boy who gnawed at his shirtsleeve our first month because he was so nervous? The boy who couldn't stop singing? I wondered if we were messing things up again by leaving. I wondered if we should just stay put.


We've been back in Maine a month now. Thorne walks around the house singing the Chinese songs from the winter musical. But I don't need him to stop. I understand the low-grade hum of anxiety in his head that compels him. It's also no surprise that Aidan is having "the sleeping problems" again. We're repeating the dislocation cycle—this time back in our home. The patterns are the same: Thorne sings, Aidan wanders the house at night and finds other people's beds to crawl into. I am the one who wonders out loud again where we are. What we've done in moving back. I can't sleep either. I've been on the lookout for Saturn but have not seen any foreboding signs. Neptune rules my house now. The novel got finished. The blank writing book Lily brought me from Italy is filled.

Last night Tony and I watched the film he'd taken of the dumpling making: Lao Wu never looks into the camera, and his hands move so fast they don't seem natural. Mao Ayi is all business too. Her hands scoop the filling into her fingers, make a small ball of it in her palm, then slide the mix into the center of the pancake, which she presses closed with her thumbs and forefingers and seals. Finished. Then on to the next one. Over and over.

Thorne laughs on camera and says, "Bui dui! Bui dui," to Lao Wu, who places his hand on Thorne's head, just for a moment. *Not okay! Not okay!* Together they whip off cookie platters of jiaozi in short minutes. Then Tony's camera follows everyone to the dining room. On film we look like some ad hoc family: two striking Chinese people—a man and a woman in their fifties with shocking black hair—chattering in Mandarin with one skinny six-year-old named Aidan and a taller version of the same boy named Thorne and their mother, who watches in quiet amazement.

"Tell us," Tony says to Mao Ayi in Mandarin on the film, "what you are eating?"

"Jiaozi," she replies clearly, and then blushes and looks away.

"Hao chi!" Aidan yells and puts a dumpling in his mouth with his chopsticks.

It hit me in my living room in Maine that we *were* a family—six people sitting around a wooden table in Beijing, sharing a lunch after spending most of the last few years together. "Look, Tony," I said and reached for his arm. "Everyone is talking in Chinese, even me." Then Thorne pops up on the camera sitting on Lao Wu's lap. Lao Wu is grinning. Beaming. He casually puts his arm on Thorne's shoulder—then his hand on Thorne's knee. Thorne leans into his chest and laughs.

Three hours later, Lao Wu drove us to the airport and asked me when we'd be coming back to China, even though we both knew it was a question I couldn't answer. "Wo bu zhi dao," I said. *Don't know.* We'd found him a job with a British family who'd just moved to Beijing. Mao Ayi would start on Monday with a family from Australia.

Lao Wu nodded at the road and responded very clearly in English, "Not good. This is not good."

Then he parked the van in international departures and he cried. So then Tony cried. And then I cried. Lao Wu had packed us a care package: more apples and bananas and pears than we could ever eat on a thirteen-hour flight to Chicago. Plus two dozen lollipops and a box of Chinese malt balls. I took the food from Lao Wu and did not try to hug him. I put my hand up in a frozen wave. The boys ran out of the van and clamped on to Lao Wu's waist. He patted their heads with his open hands and wiped his tears and patted their heads some more.

Then the boys were off just as quickly. They had luggage carts to push. An important flight to catch. They were going home, they called to him in Chinese. *Women hui jia.* And they paused to wave back at him one more time, just before the revolving glass doors swallowed them whole.

This morning during breakfast before school, I asked the boys what they missed most about China. Without pausing they both said "Lao Wu" at the same time. His absence felt palpable. What I recall most is the way he would get a quick hug in when he lifted Aidan out of the van. And the way Thorne would lean into Lao Wu's shoulder from the backseat once the van had stopped. We can't hold an entire country in our hearts or heads—so what we seem to be doing is holding certain people.

We ate our Honey Nut Cheerios then and made a list of things that were different between the United States and China. Thorne said, "School is less stressful in America," which seemed like a good thing to me.

Aidan said, "The trees are greener here, and write down that I already can't remember the playground in China." They both wanted me to add the fact that they have a new Chinese teacher in Maine who's getting them to write a rap song in Mandarin. There were no rap songs in Chinese class in Beijing.

I put the pen down and dug into my cereal. "We'll go back," I said. "Back to China for vacations and who knows." I looked over at Tony.

"Shanghai?" he said, like a question. Then he took a sip of coffee and rested his hand on my cheek and smiled. He smiles more often now than he did the last time we lived here. He's brought that ease he knew in China back with him to the States. And he talks in Mandarin on the phone all day. His new job will take him to China every other month. "I think the next place we should live is Shanghai," he repeated, laughing.

The one thing I'd like to put on our list is the part about how the last time I lived in this house I didn't have cancer. I used to actively avoid cancer news if it drifted my way. I used to change the dial on the radio station. It was as if the country called cancer didn't exist. And I miss her sometimes—that version of myself. God, she seems young to me now, though we weren't even gone three full years. That woman who guarded the good times vigilantly, even maniacally. That new mother who thought she and her kids would live forever if she could just get them to sleep more.

Strange as this may sound, I'm also relieved to find out she doesn't live in this house any longer. Someone a little stronger has taken her place. I know now that keeping bad news at bay doesn't mean bad news isn't going to come for you. And that I can still hold my heart open even if it does come. I've let go of the metaphor I'd been carrying with me all these months—I can see that cancer doesn't have to be a cultural isolation. Doesn't have to be my own private China. I have no use for that comparison anymore. I've made my peace with both countries.

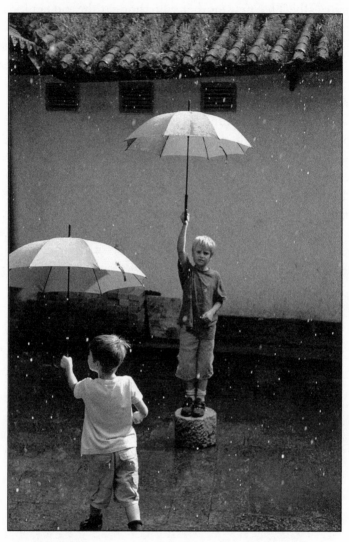

Thorne and Aidan in a sudden rainstorm in the village of
Shaxi, in Yunnan Province

# Acknowledgments

There wouldn't be as much good fortune in this story if there weren't all these people who helped. So first to my close group of writer friends: Sara Corbett, Caitlin Gutheil, Anja Hanson, Lily King, and Debra Spark. I'm indebted and humbled.

Then to my parents, Michael Conley and Thorne Conley, for their great acts of kindness and for never wavering.

To John Conley, my brother. And to Erin Conley, my sister. How lucky am I to have grown up with you two.

To the amazing Dr. Ann Partridge at Dana Farber, who inspires me every day to get out there and live. To Dr. Michelle Specht at Massachusetts General, my gratitude and respect have no end. To Dr. Celine Godin, for her wisdom and candor. To Dr. Anne Rainville for making me go back to the Beijing hospital. To Dr. Carlos Camargo for all that came after that. And to Ann, Gretchen, Jenny, Katherine, Kate, and Lisa. May we all be talking on a porch together when we're eighty.

In China, I want to thank Lao Wu, Mao Ayi, Xiao Cheng, and Rose. I'm still learning from their lessons in language and in life. Deep thanks also to the people we explored China with: Melanie Cutler and Eliot Cutler, Deb Fallows and Jim

Fallows, Lars Jorgensen, Erin Keogh and Chris Keogh, Mimi Kuo-Deemer, Molly Lloyd, Anna Poulsen, Dan Reardon, Ken Shih, Anne Stevenson-Yang, Britta Von Lewinksi, Hans Von Lewinski, Vanessa Wang, and Robyn Wexler. At the boys' school, I am so grateful to Julie Lawton, principal extraordinaire, and a group of amazing teachers: Diba Kader, Detra Watson, Amy Carlson, and Carmel Byrne.

Back in the States, I bow down to the friends and family who sent us off to China and then helped us out when things got dicey: to Annie Anderson, Jenepher Burton, Ania Camargo, my cousin Jennifer Chittick, Tyler Clements, Don Cohon, Jenna Conley, Jane Conover, Paige Cox, Sara Crisp, my cousins Elisabeth Dekker and Hans Dekker, my aunt Lynne Dekker, Becky Dilworth, Susannah Dubois, Rich Dubois, Mary Fitzgerald, Jon Fitzgerald, Maribeth Hourihan, Patty Howells, Celine Kuhn, Chris Kuhn, Winky Lewis, Monty Lewis, Katie Longstreth, Jill McGowan, Alex Millspaugh, Sarah Moran, Genevieve Morgan, Tom Morgan, Jos Nicholas, Maryanne O'Hara, Nick O'Hara, Peggy Orenstein, Susan Partridge, Derek Pierce, Judith Redwine, Gillian Schair, Electa Sevier, and Sara Woolf. To the entire Kieffer family for their support, as well as to the Meisters and the Davis family. And to all the Crouters out there, and to all the Conleys for their help, especially Chrissy Wakefield for her singing and her cheerleading (literal and otherwise) all these years.

To Sara Corbett, again, for her wisdom and friendship and for building the Telling Room with me.

To Mike Paterniti for his friendship and for his Telling Room genius. Thanks for inviting Tony to drive a Ferrari across Inner Mongolia with you. It all starts there. And thank you for sharing a small bit of your writing brilliance so I could find my way to this book.

# Acknowledgments

To Lily King, this time for her knowingness and her great friendship. I am so grateful.

To Carole Baron, for her incredible insights and her joy in the process and for understanding all parts of this journey. It has been my deepest pleasure to work with her. Thank you also to Emily Milder at Knopf for her amazing smarts and savvy; to Pat Johnson, for her intuition and support; and to Gabrielle Brooks, Lydia Buechler, and Erinn Hartman; I have been so fortunate to work with each of them.

Stephanie Cabot makes talking about writing one of the world's greatest delights. I am so lucky.

And then to the boys, Aidan and Thorne. This book has always been for them and to them. May I always be able to ask them if they know how much. And here at the end, to Tony Kieffer, for everything. And for making it all so much fun.

POSTCARDS FROM TOMORROW SQUARE
*Reports from China*
by Jame Fallows

Since December 2006, *The Atlantic Magazine*'s James Fallows has been writing some of the most discerning accounts of the economic and political transformation occurring in China. The ten essays collected here cover a wide-range of topics: from visionary tycoons and TV-battling entrepreneurs, to environmental pollution and how China subsidizes our economy. Fallows expertly and lucidly explains the economic, political, social, and cultural forces at work turning China into a world superpower at breakneck speed. This eye-opening and cautionary account is essential reading for all concerned not only with China's but America's future role in the world.

Current Affairs

WILD GRASS
*Three Stories of Change in Modern China*
by Ian Johnson

In *Wild Grass*, Pulitzer Prize—winning journalist Ian Johnson tells the stories of three ordinary Chinese citizens moved to extraordinary acts of courage: a peasant legal clerk who filed a class-action suit on behalf of overtaxed farmers, a young architect who defended the rights of dispossessed homeowners, and a bereaved woman who tried to find out why her elderly mother had been beaten to death in police custody. Representing the first cracks in the otherwise seamless façade of Communist Party control, these small acts of resistance demonstrate the unconquerable power of the human conscience and prophesy an increasingly open political future for China.

Current Affairs

VINTAGE BOOKS AND ANCHOR BOOKS
Available at your local bookstore, or visit
www.randomhouse.com

**Meet with Interesting People**
**Enjoy Stimulating Conversation**
**Discover Wonderful Books**

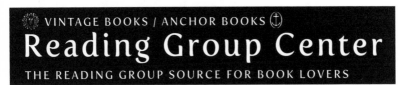

VINTAGE BOOKS / ANCHOR BOOKS

# Reading Group Center

THE READING GROUP SOURCE FOR BOOK LOVERS

Visit ReadingGroupCenter.com where you'll find great
reading choices—award winners, bestsellers, beloved
classics, and many more—and extensive resources
for reading groups such as:

## Author Chats

Exciting contests offer reading groups
the chance to win one-on-one phone
conversations with Vintage and Anchor
Books authors.

## Extensive Discussion Guides

Guides for over 450 titles as well as
non–title specific discussion questions
by category for fiction, nonfiction,
memoir, poetry, and mystery.

## Personal Advice and Ideas

Reading groups nationwide share ideas,
suggestions, helpful tips, and anecdotal
information. Participate in the discussion
and share your group's experiences.

## Behind the Book Features

Specially designed pages which can include
photographs, videos, original essays, notes
from the author and editor, and book-related
information.

## Reading Planner

Plan ahead by browsing upcoming
titles, finding author event schedules,
and more.

## Special for Spanish-language
reading groups

**www.grupodelectura.com**
A dedicated Spanish-language content
area complete with recommended titles
from Vintage Español.

### A selection of some favorite reading group titles from our list

*Atonement* by Ian McEwan
*Balzac and the Little Chinese Seamstress*
  by Dai Sijie
*The Blind Assassin* by Margaret Atwood
*The Devil in the White City* by Erik Larson
*Empire Falls* by Richard Russo
*The English Patient* by Michael Ondaatje
*A Heartbreaking Work of Staggering Genius*
  by Dave Eggers
*The House of Sand and Fog* by Andre Dubus III
*A Lesson Before Dying* by Ernest J. Gaines

*Lolita* by Vladimir Nabokov
*Memoirs of a Geisha* by Arthur Golden
*Midnight in the Garden of Good and Evil*
  by John Berendt
*Midwives* by Chris Bohjalian
*Push* by Sapphire
*The Reader* by Bernhard Schlink
*Snow* by Orhan Pamuk
*An Unquiet Mind* by Kay Redfield Jamison
*Waiting* by Ha Jin
*A Year in Provence* by Peter Mayle